POISON!

POISON!
The World's Greatest True Murder Stories

Selected, with an Introduction, by
RICHARD GLYN JONES

A STAR BOOK
published by
the Paperback Division of
W.H. Allen & Co. Plc

A Star Book
Published in 1988
by the Paperback Division of
W.H. Allen & Co Plc
44 Hill Street, London W1X 8LB

First published in Great Britain
by Xanadu Publications Ltd in 1987

Printed and bound in Great Britain by
Anchor Brendon Ltd, Tiptree, Essex

ISBN 0 352 32178 4

CONTENTS

Introduction

It takes no great act of imagination to realize that poison is as old as humanity, and that primitive man must have discovered by literally bitter experience which berries and fungi could be safely eaten, and which not. And, being human as well as primitive, it would not have been long before he began to use the lethal vegetables for his own purposes: for poisoning the tips of his spears and arrows on the one hand, and for quietly murdering his enemies on the other. Indeed, the earliest records that have survived describe trials for murder by this means, and poison has been mankind's deadly companion ever since.

The first famous poisoning was that of Socrates in 399 BC — the wisest man in Greece, according to the Delphic Oracle. A hideously ugly old fellow who had been a soldier earlier in life, he became the most influential philosopher of the ancient world, despite dressing in rags and teaching in the streets. His message was delivered not by lecturing but by rigorous questioning of his listeners, and his teachings were full of scepticism about the sciences, about the government, and — fatally — about the gods. When Athens lost the Peloponnesian war its leaders wanted a scapegoat and Socrates, with his dangerous teachings, seemed the ideal candidate. Since any citizen could bring another to trial on suspicion of a crime merely by announcing it, Socrates was quickly arrested and charged with blasphemy and corruption of the young. He was tried by a jury of no less than 501 citizens, and — no orator — spoke rather badly in his own defence, with the result that the verdict went against him 281-220. During the debate about what his punishment should be, Socrates was extremely sarcastic about his accusers, suggesting that a suitable penalty for these so-called crimes would be for them to elect him to one of the highest offices of the state and maintain him at public expense for the rest of his life. He was promptly sentenced to death. The means of his execution turned out to be the now-famous cup of hemlock, which killed him almost immediately.

Hemlock is a common enough plant on lawns and in woods, and the variety that killed Socrates was a type called poison hemlock, a surprisingly lethal member of the parsley family, which often destroys sheep and cattle, as well as people. Most of the early poisoners used vegetable poisons like this, including the one who killed the Emperor Claudius — although there is some controversy about which poison it was.

Readers of Robert Graves' two books about Claudius or viewers of the TV series will not need to be reminded of the web of intrigue and corruption that surrounded and infested the court of Ancient Rome, and most authorities agree that the poisoning was engineered by Claudius's wife Agrippina. She had recently persuaded Claudius to adopt her son from a former marriage and name him joint heir to the vast Roman Empire, alongside the son that Claudius had had by Messalina. Agrippina was now scheming to oust Claudius's own son from the succession, feeling (quite apart from any motherly concern) that if *her* son became Emperor she would be the power behind the throne, safe in his gratitude and immensely powerful in her own right.

Complicated in theory, Agrippina's plan proved difficult in practice, and fearing that her manoeuvring must have aroused Claudius's suspicions, she changed tactics and decided to get rid of *him* first. The Emperor was partial to mushrooms, and in the dish that was served there was a particularly large and juicy one. Agrippina made sure that Claudius took it. She may have doctored it herself, or may have persuaded the eunuch Halotus, the official food taster, to administer the poison, which in turn may have been prepared by the vile Locusta, recently sentenced for poisoning but who survived to enjoy a long and evil career of her own. The idea was to use a poison that would have a delayed effect, so that the murder would not be too obvious — and Locusta was exactly the person to advise about that. In any event, Claudius ate the poisoned mushroom, but he had (as usual) been drinking heavily, and he vomited up the entire contents of his stomach. Problem. If he survived there would be hell to pay, so drastic action had to be taken. Agrippina summoned the Emperor's doctor Xenophon — also in league with her — who according to one version of the story pretended to assist the vomiting with a feather, dipping this into another, stronger poison, which finished Claudius off. In another version, the deadly dose was administered in the form of an enema.

Claudius was dead, but he had died too soon, so there followed a grim pantomime in which a troupe of entertainers was brought in, who performed through the night to the dead Emperor to give the impression to those outside that things were as normal. Despite these departures from schedule, the plan worked and Agrippina's son did indeed become Emperor of the Roman Empire: he was the appalling Nero.

The mushrooms of which Claudius was so fond are now named after him — *Amanita caesaria* — and Robert Graves in 'New Light on an Old Murder' argues convincingly that the poison was the the juice of another mushroom from the same family, *Aminita phalloides* (not difficult to guess what this is named after!), which is in season at the same time as the *caesaria*, plentiful around Rome, and which does not produce any effects until several hours after it has been taken but then is invariably fatal — barring attacks of vomiting, of course. The poison that Xenophon administered, Graves believed to have come from the wild gourd, which crops up in the Bible (II Kings 4:38-41), but this is much less certain, the only evidence for it being a possible pun made some time afterwards by the satirist Seneca.

By the time of the Borgias, Rome was at the height of her Renaissance glory, but behaviour in the courts was, if anything, even more savage. The advance of knowledge meant that, even if the Philosopher's Stone was proving elusive, there was at least a degree of chemical knowledge and the ability to distil and synthesize artificial poisons, while the unscrupulousness of the nobles provided ample employment for them.

The name Borgia has become synonymous with poison, but firm evidence from these times is scarce, and it has been suggested that the notorious poison rings and phials may well have been designed to contain perfume rather than poison (very necessary in those unhygienic times), and one author wrote a lengthy book about the Borgias without using the word 'poison' once — but this was the highly eccentric Baron Corvo, so perhaps one should not make too much of that. The situation was, though, a strange one. The Borgias were a Spanish family, bitterly resented in Rome but extremely capable and immensely ambitious, and their main objective at this time was to elect a Spanish pope. In 1492, after many years of working his way up through the echelons, Roderigo Borgia became Pope Alexander VI.

He had three children by a highly-placed courtesan; illegitimate, but always acknowledged and, as they grew older, accepted into the fiercely loyal Borgia family. The two boys, Cesare and Juan, and their sister Lucrezia were in their teens when Roderigo became Pope. During their childhood they had witnessed the savagery and brutality of the times — public rapes in the streets, orgies indoors — and began to do it for themselves as soon as they were able, the two boys competing for young Lucrezia's favours. She preferred to let Cesare win. Now, at the age of sixteen, the depraved and already vicious Cesare was appointed Archbishop of Valencia, while back at Rome more and more Spaniards were put into key positions in the Vatican. It was not long before Lucrezia was married off to Giovanni Sforza, who must have been rather miffed when she was declared too young for the marriage to be consummated. Juan was the favourite of his father, Pope Alexander, however, and was given command of his armies, while Cesare itched with frustrated ambition and with jealousy over Lucrezia's marriage. But Juan failed as a military leader, Alexander engineered Lucrezia's return to Rome (Sforza heading for the hills at the prospect of a confrontation), and it was not long before Cesare began to assert himself. If he did use poison, that was only one of his techniques: stabbings, midnight abductions and mysterious drownings all played their part in his ruthless progress to power. Juan, indeed, was one of the ones dredged out of the Tiber, and the fact that the Pope ordered no investigation of the murder left little doubt as to its perpetrator. But to what extent is the Borgias' reputation as poisoners supported? The rumour was that their knowledge came from the Spanish Moors, and that they experimented and refined their venoms so that they actually improved the flavour of food and wine — but no-one knew what the Borgia poison was.

It was called *cantarella* and, according to tradition was a white powder resembling sugar but tasteless in itself. This would suggest that it was some form of arsenic. In the reign of terror that Alexander and Cesare inflicted, many of their opponents and rivals certainly died under odd circumstances, but proof in the modern sense is lacking in any specific case. The *sort* of thing that happened would be that Alexander would appear to show favour to a certain up-and-coming Cardinal — Cardinal Mihiel is a case in point — allowing him to prosper, gathering wealth and property, then craftily poisoning him; the law was that all the estates would then accrue to the Pope, and Alexander collected 150,000 ducats after Cardinal Mihiel's sudden demise. The Borgias may also have used a poison calling *aqua Toffana*, an arsenic solution developed by a Neopolitan woman named Toffana for removing skin blemishes, whose lethal properties were soon discovered by the women who bought it. The stuff had quite a vogue, quite apart from any use the Borgias may have made of it, and it is said that more than 600 husbands and elderly relatives died before it was banned.

One man who claimed to know the secret of the Borgias' venom was a villain called Exili, an Italian who at the time we meet him (1654) was languishing in the depths of the Bastille. After weeks and months of solitude and starvation, the door of the cell opened and another prisoner was flung in, a young nobleman who was by no means happy to be there. He was the Chevalier Jean Baptiste de Sainte-Croix, and he had been arrested at the request of his mistress's father, who did not approve of the *affaire*. In a strange echo of Athenian practice, it was possible in seventeenth-century France for those close to the King to have anyone arrested merely by asking.

This mistress was Madame de Brinvilliers, and her father's disapproval of the liaison is understandable, for ever since her marriage she had been carrying on quite openly with a variety of lovers, and although Sainte-Croix was more constant than most, he was a notorious scoundrel in his own right. Nonetheless, the young Chevalier was full of thoughts of revenge, and when Exili revealed that he was a master-poisoner and willing to share some of his secrets, he found an eager listener. The Borgia poison, it seemed, involved feeding some concoction to a bear, hanging it upside down, and collecting the saliva or vital juices somehow or other... Three months later, Sainte-Croix was released and lost no time in returning to Madame, no doubt telling her of his new-found skills at the earliest opportunity. She too proved an interested audience, and in no time at all they had decided to poison her father, possibly for revenge, but principally so that they would be free of his interference and comfortably provided for by his estate. By an unfortunate coincidence her father was at that moment taken ill, which provided the Marquise with a perfect opportunity to go to the country and 'nurse' him.

Sainte-Croix provided the poison from his new laboratory (whether it contained a bear we are not told); the old man ate a poisoned meal, and he died after four days of internal agony, the country doctors suspecting nothing more than indigestion. Easy!

Sainte-Croix soon fancied himself a master-poisoner, and Madame was becoming thoughtful as they whipped through her father's inheritance at whirlwind speed. If it wasn't for her brothers and her sister, how much more she would have had... It was necessary to be cautious, however, as a spate of similar deaths might arouse suspicions, so Madame decided to carry out a few scientific tests. The first experiment was on her maid, who received a dose of the brew and immediately suffered acute pains, but she was saved by a doctor applying an emetic. Clearly, more tests had to be made. Madame promptly presented herself as a volunteer at the large hospital nearby, ministering to the patients with her new 'medicine'. Very soon the doctors were faced with a mysterious epidemic of a strange lethargy that seized the inmates and quickly killed them. Autopsies revealed nothing suspicious. Madame, callously murdering dozens of such victims, now knew the exact dosages needed, and that the poison was for all practical purposes undetectable.

The two brothers were quickly despatched. The sister managed to escape, but Madame de Brinvilliers had by now developed a taste for poisoning. There was no longer any question of gain. She may have liked the power it gave her, or just liked it for its own sake, but, either way, she was picking off victims indiscriminately. Sometimes they were lovers with whom she was bored, while others were simply people who annoyed her in some trifling way: one died for spilling coffee on her dress. Her husband also received his share of poison, but Sainte-Croix — not the marrying kind — always managed to provide an antidote. But dozens of people did die, and it might have gone on for years but for an unfortunate accident. Sainte-Croix wore a glass face-mask to ward off the noxious fumes while he experimented, but one day the mask slipped and the Chevalier was overcome. The servant who discovered his body panicked and, Madame being out, summoned the authorities. They seized Sainte-Croix's notes and papers, and Madame, realizing that the game was up, fled to England, then to Germany, then on to a convent in Liege, where she wrote a lengthy confession of her sins — but her hideout was discovered and she was brought back to Paris for trial. Her confession proved her own guilt, but she refused to reveal her accomplices and was tortured in an attempt to get her to name them; one of the tortures, which involved stretching the Marquise over a trestle and pouring large quantities of water into her mouth, is depicted in the charming frontispiece to this book. 'All that water for such a little woman as I!', she remarked, and told them nothing. Her courage brought her a good deal of respect, but it did not stop her being beheaded and burned a short time afterwards. Nor did her execution stop the general craze for poisoning, in what has been called 'The Age of Arsenic'.

It was again the Italians who inspired Thomas Griffiths Wainewright. He quit the army complaining that the colours of the uniforms were too harsh, and attempted to pursue a career in art and letters. He might have succeeded, too, for his paintings were admired by Blake and his prose was praised by Lamb, Hazlitt and De Quincey, whom he got to know and whose company he craved. The problem was that the artistic collections and the little gatherings cost money, which an annuity of £200 could not support, and his artistic endeavours — successful as they were — did not add appreciably to this total. He therefore asked the four trustees who controlled his money whether he could realize the capital from which this annual interest accrued and, in the face of their flat refusal, decided to employ his artistic talents on a likeness of their signatures. The Bank of England coughed up without demur, and a criminal career was launched.

The £2259 helped things along for a while, but those tedious creditors were soon threatening to interrupt the little *soirées* once more. Forgery would not work a second time (in this context, anyway), but there was an uncle with a fine house and a very decent income — and, alas, excellent health. During his study of classical Italian literature, Wainewright had come across a pamphlet on poisons, and the glamour of the whole business had fascinated him; a sensitive soul such as his would have recoiled from the idea of violence, but a subtle poison in uncle's wine? It was easily done, and Wainewright was soon installed in Linden House with his wife and child. The extravagant living continued and, while some of the creditors were paid off, others soon appeared, as did Wainewright's mother-in-law plus two daughters by a second marriage, who moved in to share the Wainewrights' good fortune.

There were rumours that he now began to use his artistic influence to pass off spurious engravings as genuine, but this was chickenfeed: much more substantial funds were needed if the dilettante life was to continue, so Wainewright hatched a plot to insure the lives of all these in-laws, in particular sister-in-law Helen. There was a cunning touch in that Helen's life was insured in sister Madeleine's name, from whom Wainewright knew he would be able to extract money; the arrangements were completed over the Christmas week of 1830, and Helen ceased to exist shortly afterwards. When her mother began asking questions about Helen's death, she was poisoned too. But when Madeleine tried to claim the £18,000 insurance there were problems, and creditors were presenting even more pressing problems, and so finally Wainewright was obliged to abandon his literary life and flee to the continent, where he hid for several years. He eventually returned to England in disguise and hoped that he would avoid capture, but by now he was universally known as Wainewright the Poisoner and his arrest followed rapidly. In Newgate he became something of a celebrity (when taxed with the murder of pretty young Helen, he pointed out that 'she had very thick ankles'), but he was sentenced to transportation and died lonely and neglected in Tasmania.

His writings are no longer read, and Wainewright's only real contribution to the literature for which he strived so hard was to inspire a splendid essay from that other wit, Oscar Wilde.

The long age of indiscriminate poisoning was now drawing to a close. Huge advances were being made in toxicology, and those potions once thought undetectable could now be traced fairly easily — but poisons were still very easily available to anyone who wanted them, and offered a temptation to the unscrupulous. The career of William Palmer shows the sort of callousness that we have come to recognize in wholesale poisoners, and ushers in the modern era of poisoning which is documented in this book. The son of a weak father and a domineering mother, Palmer had a conventional Victorian upbringing with lots of church on Sundays and lots of study during the week, but as soon as he went to London to study medicine he abandoned the churchgoing and cultivated all sorts of bad habits. On qualifying, he took up a practice in the country town of Rugely and his financial problems seemed to be solved when he married a wealthy wife.

Palmer's career resembles Wainewright's in some respects — although it is drastically different in others. Where Wainewright had needed money to support his artistic pretensions, Palmer needed it to finance his speculations on horses, which were wild and extravagant. Known and liked as a jolly fellow on every racecourse, Palmer's gambling schemes were regarded with dismay by those who actually knew what they were doing, and before long the creditors were gathering. His wife's money, it turned out, was not freely available to Palmer but doled out in quarterly instalments, so — like Wainewright — he needed to get his hands on some capital. Just as the financial situation was getting drastic, Palmer's wife died of 'bilious cholera' and he lost no time in claiming the insurance money. This kept things ticking over for a while, but — the familiar story — as the money was swallowed up on the track the idea of a repeat performance suggested itself. The candidate this time was Palmer's brother George, and he soon died of the same mysterious complaint, but this time the insurance company was suspicious and refused to pay up. If Palmer had been able to turn back, this would have been the moment to do it, but his gambling debts were enormous and *something* had to be done;

he found another victim in John Parsons Cook, a fellow gambler whom he had been cheating for some time and who was now asking awkward questions. He also happened to possess a large sum of money. His death would solve three problems, by fending off awkward inquiries, cancelling the debts he owed to Cook, and presenting Palmer with a sizeable sum for himself. In fact, it solved none of them, for Cook's death immediately turned what had been mere suspicion into action, and Palmer was arrested.

The bodies of Palmer's wife and his brother were exhumed, and examined for strychnine. It was not detected — but it must quickly be added that the examination was a farce, with Palmer bribing the postmaster to show him the analysis report, and attempting to bribe the messenger bringing some of the organs to 'accidentally' smash the jar which contained them. Palmer's trial attracted the attention of the whole nation and he was found guilty on circumstantial evidence. Just before he was hanged he remarked, 'It's the riding that's done it'.

The poisoners collected in the pages that follow include most of the famous names from the modern period (meaning the last 150 years or so), together with some lesser-known though equally interesting practitioners. The most notable omission is Florence Bravo, who has already appeared in one of these collections*, but here you will meet Mrs Maybrick, Adelaide Bartlett, Jessie Costello and Madeleine Smith amongst the ladies, and Doctors Cream, Crippen, Waite and Pritchard amongst the men. (Poison has been called the cowards' weapon and also the ladies' weapon; there would seem to be an equally good case for calling it the doctors' weapon.) If arsenic seems to predominate, that is because it has been far and away the most popular of all poisons, and a fair sample would probably include an even greater proportion of such cases — but I have tried to show as wide a variety as possible of both poison and poisoners. They form an interesting collection, for of all murderers it is the poisoners who are in many ways the most fascinating characters, and it is always the human personality that makes crime worth reading about.

— R.G.J

*Unsolved! Classic True Murder Cases (London: Xanadu, 1987)

JOHN DUNNING
Murder and the Mother Superior

The three young women standing in front of the charge desk in the squad room of the Wetteren police station were nuns and the desk sergeant knew them by sight, if not by name.

Wetteren is, after all, a small place. Located roughly ten miles to the east of Ghent, Belgium and a little to the north of the main highway running from Brussels to Ostend, it is a quiet community of under twenty thousand souls with a small shopping centre, seven catholic churches, thirty-one taverns, a brothel and an old people's home. There is a cloister next to the Old People's Home which houses not only the nursing sisters, but also those engaged in teaching and other activities.

'Yes?' said the sergeant politely. He was intrigued over what might have brought three nuns to the police station. If there had been a burglary at the cloister, someone could have simply telephoned or, even if it had been felt that the report should be made in person, one nun would have sufficed. Why three?

To his astonishment, there was no immediate answer. The three nuns looked nervously at each other as if each was waiting for the others to speak and said nothing.

The sergeant cleared his throat. It was a Monday morning, January 16, 1978, and he was not feeling exactly at his most cheerful. Wetteren lies in the heart of Flanders and the weather was, of course, rotten, a grey, gloomy, depressing day with bitterly cold showers of mixed rain and hail sweeping one after another over the city.

'We think we want to report a murder,' blurted one of the nuns abruptly, her voice a squeak of nervous excitement and embarrassment.

The sergeant opened his mouth and then shut it again without saying anything. He did not know what to say. It was over thirty years since

15

there had been a homicide in Wetteren. It occurred to him that the woman might be drunk or playing a practical joke, but how could that be? They were nuns.

'You mean you don't know whether you want to report it or not?' he asked cautiously.

'No, no!' said another nun. 'We mean we want to report what we think is a murder. Maybe it isn't. We hope it isn't.'

'Very well,' said the sergeant resignedly. 'Who has been murdered?'

'We think Mrs Maria van der Gunst,' said the nun who had spoken first. 'She was a patient at the Old People's Home.'

'She has just died?' asked the sergeant, his finger poised over the dial of the internal communication system.

'Oh no,' said the nun. 'She died on the fifth of July last year.'

The sergeant stared at her with a total lack of comprehension and then dialled.

'Franz?' he said into the telephone. 'Is the inspector there yet? Listen. I have what appears to be a report on a homicide. Could you come down and talk to the people? Would you do it right now? Right. I'll make out an F.I.R., if you think that's best.'

He hung up the telephone.

'Someone from the Department of Criminal Investigations will be down immediately,' he said. He took a printed First Information Report form out of the drawer of the desk. 'Now, may I have your names please?'

The nuns turned out to be named Franziska, Godlive and Pieta. They were all members of the Order of Holy Joseph living in the cloister and working in the Old People's Home. They were young, shy and looked remarkably innocent.

The story which they had to tell was, however, anything but innocent and the sergeant found it so shocking and improbable that his pen hung suspended and motionless over the form as he sat literally paralyzed, his mouth hanging open in astonishment.

According to the charges that the nuns wished, however reluctantly, to file, the murderess was the Mother Superior of their order and the directress of the Old People's Home.

The only conclusion that the sergeant could reach was that, for some unexplained reason, the three young nuns had gone insane simultaneously. He knew Sister Godfrida, the Mother Superior, by sight, a sturdy, stern-looking woman in her mid-forties and he knew that she had been at the convent for close to thirty years. She was not only the last person in the world to be suspected of murdering her patients; there was also no reason in the world why she would want to.

He was, therefore, on the point of summoning a doctor to take the poor, insane nuns away when Detective-Sergeant Franz Gropa came down from the Department of Criminal Investigations and did so.

Upstairs in the office of Inspector Dyke Van Horn, the nuns repeated their charge with much the same effect as they had had in the charge room below.

'But why?' said the inspector, his eyes bulging slightly. 'Why in the name of Heaven would she do such a thing?'

He was a stocky man, somewhat under average height, with a high, broad, forehead and his brown eyes were abnormally deep-set. Having been involved in criminal investigations for nearly twenty years, he had thought that he had heard everything. Now, he realized that he had not, but he still had no idea of how much more he still had to hear.

The three nuns looked at each other again, their faces mirroring an inner struggle.

'We are sinning,' said Sister Godlive. 'There is a vow of silence on us.'

'Put on us by the director,' said Sister Franziska. 'But he is not our superior in the church.'

'Sister Godfrida is, said Sister Pieta.

'Her sins are greater than ours,' said Sister Franziska.

Sister Godlive turned to the inspector.

'Sister Godfrida murdered Mrs van der Gunst because she wanted her money and jewellery,' she said.

The inspector made a mental note that she had now said that it was murder, not that she thought it was murder.

'An excellent motive for murder,' he said. 'One of the more common. But not with nuns. What would she do with the money?'

'Pay for her expensive meals in fine restaurants and for her wines and brandy,' said Sister Godlive.

'Buy her filthy pornographic magazines and her sex toys,' said Sister Pieta.

'And her drugs, her morphine, her heroine, her cocaine and the other things,' said Sister Franziska.

The inspector got up from his desk, walked all around it and sat back down again. A very strong feeling of unreality had suddenly invaded his prosaic, somewhat shabby office. Expensive restaurants? Wines? Pornography! Sex toys!! MURDER!!! In the convent of the Old People's Home?

Sergeant Gropa, a normally rather handsome, young man with an open, good-natured face and short-cut blond hair, was sitting at his desk with mouth and eyes wide open, looking like an idiot. Abruptly, he closed his mouth.

'Loudun!' he said opening it again.

The inspector considered the idea, eyeing the nuns a little warily. He was, of course, familiar with the case of possession or, depending upon your outlook, collective hysteria which had taken place in Loudun, France, and which had been made famous in the book *The Devils of Loudun*. There, an entire convent of nuns had gone into a sort of sexual frenzy, exhibiting their private parts to the gaze of the idly curious, and demanding sexual satisfaction on the spot. Had the Devil come to Wetteren?

If so, it was for a different form of manifestation. The young nuns showed no incline to fling themselves on the floor and display their genitals. Rather, all three were pink with embarrassment.

So was the inspector and he got up again and went to gaze out of the window so that he could put his questions with his back turned.

'If what you claim is true,' he said slowly, 'this must have been going on for some time. Why do you come to us only now?'

'Because she came back,' said Sister Franziska.

'She was sent away to be cured of her drug addiction last year,' said Sister Godlive. 'But at Christmas we received a postcard from her. It said, "I shall soon be with you." We didn't believe it, but last Friday she came back and now it has all started again.'

'You mean your superiors knew that Sister Godfrida was a drug addict?' said the inspector. 'Do they know that you have come to the police?'

'No,' said Sister Pieta. 'In fact, we were specifically forbidden to speak of these matters outside the convent. Everyone there knows about Sister Godfrida and what she is doing, but no one can say anything because we are sworn to silence. They say that the reputation of the order must be preserved at all costs.'

'But we have talked it over among ourselves,' said Sister Godlive, 'and we decided that our vows are to the Church and to God. What Sister Godfrida is doing is an offence to God and, even if our superiors forbids us, we should disobey and try to stop her before she kills still more of the old people.'

'You are suggesting that she has killed others besides Mrs van der Gunst?' asked the inspector.

'Yes,' said Sister Godlive. 'Many others perhaps. This has been going on for nearly seven years. Ever since she had her brain operation.'

For the first time since the nuns had entered the office, the inspector began to have a feeling that this conversation was not, perhaps, as insane as it sounded. Sister Godfrida had had a brain operation. Perhaps it had left her deranged in some manner or other. It was, at least, possible. Otherwise, the whole story made no sense. You did not become the Mother Superior of a convent if you were on hard drugs and addicted to gourmet foods, expensive wines and pornography.

'Very well,' he said. 'How do you think that Sister Godfrida murdered Mrs van Der Gunst?'

'She gave her an overdose of insulin,' said Sister Franziska without hesitation. 'She was an old woman, eighty-seven, and she had diabetes. Even if there had been an autopsy, it would not have shown anything because she had been receiving insulin anyway, but there was no autopsy, of course.'

'I don't know if an autopsy now would show anything or not,' said the inspector. 'I would like you to speak with our medical expert. Do you mind if I call him?'

The inspector wanted Dr Fons Shryker's opinion on whether an overdose of insulin would show up in an autopsy, but he also wanted him to meet and speak to the three nuns. What they had been saying was so incredible that the possibility that they themselves were on drugs could not be excluded.

Dr Shryker, a slender, elegant sort of man with rimless spectacles and a small moustache, came to the inspector's office, confirmed that an overdose of insulin could probably not be determined in the autopsy of a person who had been taking insulin in any case and certainly not when the victim had been buried for close to half a year, expressed the opinion that they were not only sane, but telling the literal truth in so far as they knew it.

'But, my God!' said the inspector in dismay. 'This is a terrible case for us to handle. How can I go to the Prosecutor and tell him that I want to investigate the Mother Superior of the convent because she is mudering the patients in order to spend their money on gourmet meals, fine wines, sex toys, drugs and pornography? Even if he doesn't send me for psychiatric observation, how would we ever prove such things?'

'If it's true, she must be clinically insane,' said the sergeant. 'Wouldn't a psychiatric examination show that? Even if we couldn't prove homicide, we could at least get her committed to some institution where she would be out of harm's way.'

'You couldn't force her to submit to a psychiatric examination.' said the doctor. 'She'd have to cooperate and, in any case, I'm not certain that you could get her committed purely on the basis of the examination and the accusations of three nuns.'

'I'm sure we couldn't,' said the inspector, 'because, if they're telling the truth, then the Order would do everything possible to cover the thing up. They wouldn't cooperate and, even if she would, they wouldn't let her.'

'Then what do we do?' said the sergeant. 'We can't simply forget about it. Those nuns have lodged an official complaint, even if there's no F.I.R. on it. We have to take some action.'

'I'm quite aware of that,' said the inspector a little testily. 'We will take action, but, at the moment, I don't know what action to take. Maybe we could start by making a very discreet investigation of the charges. See what you can do with that, but handle it personally. I don't want a word of this to get out.'

Sergeant Gropa was a well-trained and clever investigator, but he had no easy task in assembling background material on Sister Godfrida without anyone in Wetteren suspecting that he was doing so. She was, after all, a rather conspicuous figure in such a small community and she had been a member of her order for twenty-nine years.

The early history was unexceptional. The daughter of a devout, lower-income family, she had entered the Order of Holy Joseph at the age of fifteen, apparently more at the wish of her parents, who lived in the neighbouring village of Overmere, than at her own. Her name had been Cécile Blombeck. She was now forty-four years old, a plump, grim-looking woman who wore rimless glasses, and most of her career had been as a nursing nun. In 1971, she had herself been operated on for a brain tumour. The operation had been a complete success.

Or had it?

For the sergeant soon began turning up reports of less banal activity following it. Sister Godfrida had been seen two years earlier at an extremely expensive restaurant in a very stylish seaside resort on the

Belgian coast with another nun, Sister Mathieu, who was considerably younger and not a nurse but a teacher. The nuns had been wearing not their habits, but chic trouser suits. Both had been more than a little drunk and had shown a tendency to fondle each other.

'Good God!' said the inspector when he had read this part of the sergeant's report. 'Don't tell me that she's a lesbian as well!'

'It appears to be a close friendship,' said the sergeant cautiously. 'I have other reports from people who spotted her in restaurants in Ghent and Brussels and, generally, she was with Sister Mathieu.'

Whether he wanted it or not, this was what the inspector needed. It was confirmation that the story told by Sisters Franziska, Godlive and Pieta was not a complete fabrication. There had been something strange in the comportment of Sister Godfrida following her operation and, if that much were true, then the rest might well be. The case which had, up until now, remained unofficial and untitled, became the 'Investigation into the Suspected Homicide of Maria van der Gunst on or about July 5, 1977'.

That grounds for suspicion of homicide existed did not solve the problem of how the police were to prove it, and it seemed to the inspector that short of a voluntary confession or being caught red-handed in a second murder there was little hope of a solution to the case.

The best he thought might be done was to assemble enough evidence of erratic conduct on the part of Sister Godfrida from the other nuns for her to be quietly removed from contact with patients in the Old People's Home and, if necessary, committed.

The only source from which he could obtain such information was, however, from persons under her authority and he was not at all sure that the others would be as willing to violate the injunction of silence laid upon them as had been Sisters Franziska, Godlive and Pieta.

There was not even any certainty that he would be able to get further statements from those three.

'I'm afraid the only way to handle this,' he told the sergeant, 'is to make an open, official case out of it, have the body exhumed and autopsied and bring in the nuns for questioning. If we're able to establish our case, we'll then proceed to the arrest and interrogation of the suspect.'

'And, if none of them talk?' asked the sergeant.

'In that case, our position will be very difficult here in Wetteren,' said the inspector.

'The population will undoubtedly consider us to be communists, atheists or insane and the Order of Holy Joseph will be forced to take legal action against us for defamation. Under the circumstances, I suspect that the commissioner would have to take action.'

'Meaning that neither of us would remain in criminal investigations,' said the sergeant in alarm. 'Why do it then? I do not like walking a beat in the factory district.'

'Because it's our job,' said the inspector. 'And besides, I may be in an old people's home myself one day. I would hope that the police would be making some effort to see that I was not murdered by drug-addicted, lesbian nuns.'

Actually, the inspector did not have much to fear even if he did end up in an old people's home, for the case of Sister Godfrida was without question unique in Belgium and probably in all Europe.

In the opinion of Dr Shryker, her case was the result of an unusual combination of circumstances which would, it was devoutly hoped, never be repeated and which had originated with the brain operation seven years earlier.

'An operation like that is a tricky thing,' he told the inspector. 'There is still not enough known about the brain, but we do know such an intervention can result in profound, if not immediately obvious, personality changes.

'This is apparently what happened with Sister Godfrida. Physically and mentally, the operation was a success, but, psychologically, it was a disaster. Certain tendencies that had been latent became dominant. Certain inhibitions were suppressed. An alteration in the psychological balance obviously took place and resulted in a woman who looked like Sister Godfrida and who had superficially the same personality, but who was, in fact, a totally different person.'

That Sister Godfrida was a different person from the one she had been before her operation was already certain, for the evidence that had now been assembled showed that prior to that time, she had been a very ordinary sort of Mother Superior at the Old People's Home. A hard worker and a strict disciplinarian, she had been considered demanding but fair, not asking more of the nurses under her than she was prepared to perform herself.

There was no hint of any improper behaviour with the other nuns or with the patients and to everyone who knew her, the thought of her indulgence in gourmet meals, expensive wines, drugs and pornography was simply laughable.

Following the operation, things had changed abruptly. Sister Godfrida had been given morphine to still the post-operative pain and it had proved, in her case, fatally addictive. She became willing to do anything to get it, and the manner in which she went about this was described in the testimony of another young nun, known as Sister Ursule.

In her statement to the police she said, 'I came to the patient's room at approximately ten o'clock in the evening. He was a man in his sixties and still vigorous.'

'Sister Godfrida was standing beside the bed and she had lifted the skirts of her habit and was showing him her body. I heard her say, 'If you pay me well, I will make you happy.'

'She then asked him for three thousand francs and he agreed. He was lying on the bed in a dressing gown and she put her hand inside of it. He also began touching her body.

'I thought that I had gone insane or was having a vision sent by the Devil, so I went back to the duty room and took a small glass of brandy to clear my head.

'This happened in the summer of 1972 or 1973 when I had not been long in the order. I did not tell anyone about it, but later on, there were many such things and Sister Godfrida would offer herself to the patients, both men and women, even if others of us were present. She did not seem to care.'

She had little reason to care. Sister Godfrida's activities were not motivated solely by commercial considerations and her fellow sisters were made the same offers gratis although 'offer' was not precisely the right term as Sister Godfrida's was not only insistent, but remained a strict disciplinarian in this respect as well.

'When we came on duty,' ran the nearly identical statements of a number of the young novices, 'Sister Godfrida would make us kneel on the floor and kiss her feet. She said she had no objection if we did it higher up. She pulled up our habits and jabbed us in the buttocks, the thighs and our private parts with a hypodermic needle. If anyone complained, she beat them with a dog whip.'

The inspector need not have feared for lack of testimony. Once the ice had been broken, the statements poured in from every side.

Sister Godfrida had consistently approached the nun on night duty with homosexual requests. Sister Godfrida had beaten nuns, novices and patients alike. Sister Godfrida had visited the younger nuns and novices in their beds and had sought to engage in lesbian relations with them.

On this last point, there was a slight disagreement. All of the Sisters insisted that they had repulsed their sex-mad superior personally, but were quite certain that the others had been forced to yield.

On another point, however, there was total unanimity and this was the almost public love-making between Sister Godfrida and Sister Mathieu and the great feasts and celebrations they had held in the convent itself. The most extravagant foods and the finest of wines were served, but only for Sisters Godfrida and Mathieu. The others were restricted to a diet of bread, boiled potatoes and water, accompanied by the comforting thought that mortification of the flesh was part of the religious experience. The patients in the Old People's Home fared no better, but, being old, had little appetite in any case.

Even taking into account the vow of silence which had been imposed on the members of the Order, it was a tribute to the nuns' devotion to their vocation that nothing had previously come out regarding the incredible goings-on in the convent and Old People's Home. The Sisters had clung loyally and desperately to their vows and it had been only the suspicion of murder which had finally brought them to speak out. As the inspector later learned, the decision to go to the police had been made by a large number of the nuns and not merely the three who had acted as spokeswomen.

From the inspector's point of view, of course, Sister Godfrida's gourmet taste, her fine wines and even her pornography and sex-toy collections were of no official interest. Even her lesbian assaults on the younger Sisters was not something on which he could take action. Theoretically, homosexuality is illegal in Belgium, but female homosexuality taking place within a convent would be extremely difficult to prove and, in any case, none of the victims was prepared to file charges, all insisting that, although others had been subjected to the most vile indignities, they themselves had escaped unscathed.

What the statements did indicate, if not prove, was that there was a basis for the accusations of murder. Obviously, for Sister Godfrida to have been murdering her patients, she would have to have been mad as a hatter and the accounts of her conduct indicated precisely that.

Even so, the inspector proceeded with the utmost caution. The descriptions of the Mother Superior's behaviour were simply incredible and he could hardly believe them himself. Supposing she denied everything and claimed that the nuns had mounted a conspiracy against her? She was known to be a strict disciplinarian. There was even a possibility that it really was no more than that, although the inspector did not believe it. There had been too many cross-references in the nuns' statements and practically no contradictions at all.

What he needed was some form of material evidence and the most likely place to look for it was in Sister Godfrida's finances. Drugs she might have been able to obtain by stealing from the elderly patients, many of whom were prescribed some kind of narcotics or others, but fine restaurants, wines, clothing and pornography all cost money. Did Sister Godfrida have any legitimate source of such funds?

It was quickly determined that she did not. There are orders which permit their members to own property, make investments and even play the stock market if they wish, but the Order of Holy Joseph was not one of them. Sister Godfrida was paid only a token salary, barely enough to buy a single second-rate pornographic magazine a month. Moreover, she did not come from a family where there was a possibility of an inheritance.

There was one other means by which she could have come into possession of money and that was by earning it by prostituting herself to the patients. But, although many of the Sisters had reported sexual activities between the Mother Superior and her charges, not all had reported seeing money change hands. In at least one case, the patient with whom Sister Godfrida had allegedly engaged in sex in one form or another was completely penniless and a charity case.

This did not, however, mean anything. Sister Godfrida's sexual exertions could not have all been commercially orientated for she had briskly pursued practically every nun in the convent and none of them had been in a position to pay for her services.

The inspector's conclusion was that Sister Godfrida was a woman who was not averse to turning a profit from sex, but if there was no money in it, she was prepared to do it for nothing.

As for earning enough from the patients to finance her exuberant life-style, it was soon shown that this would have been impossible. Few of the patients were persons of means and the majority of them were beyond the age where sexual offers, however tempting, either would or could be accepted. From statements taken from the patients later, it turned out that many had been horrified or had doubted their own sanity and had refused. The refusal had not, always been accepted. When the spirit moved her, Sister Godfrida was not a woman to take no for an answer.

The patients had been, of course, completely at her mercy and justifiably terrified of their chief nurse, for she had not hesitated to use the dog whip on them that she used on the nuns and the novices. As a matter of fact, she had used it rather more freely on the patients, as they then complained of pain and were prescribed morphine by the doctor. The morphine was, of course, appropriated for Sister Godfrida's personal use and the patients were given aspirin, if anything.

In the end, the inspector came to the conclusion that he had enough evidence to present his case and he moved to take the suspect into custody in as discreet a manner as possible. He did not think that there would be an indictment because Sister Godfrida would obviously be sent for psychological observation and he was confident that she would be declared unfit to stand trial.

Her recent conduct provided ample support for this belief. Although she had known for some time that the investigation was going on and that she herself was the object of it, she had in no way altered her behaviour and had continued beating nuns and patients, making sexual advances and living a life of luxury enjoyed by few members of the holy orders.

Whether Sister Mathieu, who had been one of the main beneficiaries of her friend's extremely modern and liberated attitudes, came to the conviction that the ball was over and that it was time to disassociate or whether the quarrel had had some other cause, the two women had engaged in a savage sort of fist fight in the convent, ripping off a scandalous amount of each other's clothing before being separated by the thunderstruck nuns. The conflict had been so violent that it had been necessary to summon a carpenter to repair the damage to the furniture.

A court order and the permission of the relatives had, in the meantime, been obtained for the exhumination of the corpse of Maria van der Gunst, but, as the doctor had feared, the subsequent autopsy failed to establish anything definite. Mrs van der Gunst had been diabetic and had been taking insulin for many years. There were traces of it in her body, but whether the quantity taken had been correct, could no longer be determined.

This troubled the inspector as there was now no evidence of homicide at all other than the unsupported statements of the nuns and, if Sister Godfrida were to prove uncooperative, it would be impossible to obtain an indictment.

He need not have worried. Whatever other failings she might have, Sister Godfrida was a truthful woman and, when asked by the inspector if she had had anything to do with the death of Maria van der Gunst, she replied, 'Yes indeed. I sent her to Heaven because she was too noisy. She disturbed my sleep.'

In response to the inspector's relieved inquiry as to how she accomplished this, she confirmed what the nuns had said and stated that she had given the old woman an overdose of insulin.

The case was, for all practice purposes, over. There had been homicide. The murderess had been identified and had confessed. It was unlikely that she would stand trial, but she could, at least, be restricted from causing any further harm.

As the inspector was, however, interested in knowing how many homicides he had solved in the case, he continued the questioning.

He did not find out and no one ever will, for only Sister Godfrida knew and she cannot remember. In two other cases, those of eighty-two-year-old Pieter Diggmann and seventy-eight-year-old Léonie Maihofer, she was certain. She had sent both of them to Heaven with insulin overdoses in February of 1977. On anything prior to that time, she was vague, but a subsequent study of the medical records and death certificates from the Old People's Home led a medical commission to believe Sister Godfrida had been responsible for approximately thirty deaths among her patients, thus assuring her a place among the great non-military, non-political mass murderers of all time.

As had been anticipated, Sister Godfrida was ordered to be sent for psychological observation, very promptly declared unfit to stand trial and quietly committed to a mental institution where she is expected to remain for the rest of her life as the psychiatrists fear that her condition is incurable.

Sister Godfrida accepted this all humbly, cheerfully and uncomplainingly, declaring herself submissive to God's will.

It was only to be expected of her. She is, after all, a nun.

Q. PATRICK
The Last of Mrs Maybrick

On 23 October 1941, in a small, woodland shack between Gaylordsville and South Kent, Connecticut, a little old woman died. It was the lonely, inconspicuous death of an obscure eighty-year-old recluse, and her body might have lain long undiscovered had it not been for a kindly neighbour whose habit it was to supply her with the milk that she needed to feed her innumerable cats.

This neighbour, peering through the fly-spotted window-pane, saw the crumpled little body lying dead amidst the filth and disarray with which, in life, she had chosen to surround herself. A cat or two, perhaps, nosing at one of the many grimy, milkless saucers, might have felt that life had changed for the worse. There was nothing or no one else to mourn the passing of this forlorn and eccentric character whom Gaylordsville and South Kent had known as Mrs Florence Chandler.

'Mrs Chandler', after a residence of twenty years, had become a familiar if somewhat shy figure in those parts, especially on the campus of the South Kent School where she was often seen, a dowdy, meagre little figure with a face wrinkled as a walnut, carrying over her spare shoulder a gunny-sack stuffed with newspapers salvaged from academic ash-cans. These newspapers comprised almost her only form of reading matter. Once she had written a book herself, but that was long ago, and South Kent School knew nothing of her as a woman of letters. Now, too poor to buy books, she was too proud to borrow them. As intellectual nourishment for her, therefore, there was nothing but old copies of the *New York Times* and an occasional *Bridgeport Sunday Post*.

'Mrs Chandler's' gunny-sack served another less literary purpose. On outgoing journeys it would often be filled with indeterminate scraps of food which were dumped at strategic points, usually on the school

28

campus, for the delectation of the neighbourhood cats. 'Mrs Chandler' had definite views on the care of cats. It was her belief that the summer folk went junketing off with the first fall of autumn leaves, leaving their cats to starve. Hence the amateur filling stations for orphaned pets.

This humanitarian impulse of 'Mrs Chandler's' was, on the whole, detrimental to the high seriousness of the South Kent students and a headache to certain members of the staff.

Headache! The word is pregnant. For when the kind neighbour discovered the pathetic body of 'Mrs Chandler' in the desolate New England shack, he had no idea that he was looking at all that remained of one of the world's greatest headaches. That tiny, dishevelled creature had, in her day, caused more headaches possibly than any woman since Helen of Troy. She had been a headache to several American Presidents; to Secretaries of State; to their wives; to many famous journalists; and to a vasty army of organized American women. She had been more than a headache to one celebrated English judge, in that she is reputed to have pushed him off the teetering brink of his sanity. Indeed, she had been a fifteen-year migraine to no less august a personage than the Queen-Empress Victoria.

And the name of that headache was Mrs Florence Maybrick.

Mrs Maybrick. To those in their carefree twenties, the name may ring a distant bell. To those in their thirties, it may conjure up dim memories of a murderess, an adulteress—or something interesting. To those over forty-five, Mrs Maybrick will be remembered for what she actually was—an international incident.

She was born Florence Chandler in Mobile, Alabama, in 1862, and came from what is usually referred to as 'good American stock', boasting among her forbears, direct and collateral, a Secretary of the Treasury, a Chief Justice, a bishop and two Episcopal rectors, co-authors of a work entitled: 'Why We Believe the Bible'. As an appendix to this illustrious list of ancestors, her mother had married, a second time, the Baron Adolph von Roques, a distinguished German officer of the Eighth Cuirassier Regiment. Little Florence was educated, partly in America, partly abroad, by a succession of the most impeccable 'masters and governesses'. Nothing had been overlooked that might insure for her a cultivated and lady-like future.

As it happened, however, these fair beginnings did not help her much, for, from an early period, Florence Chandler was dogged by bad luck. At the age of eighteen, when the other Mobile maidens of her generation were fluttering toward good clean American romance, it is reliably reported that Florence, during a rough Atlantic crossing, stumbled on the sun-deck of the liner carrying her to Europe. She stumbled and fell—literally and catastrophically—into the arms of a Cad, an English cad, at that. And, after all, the English invented the word.

The Cad was James Maybrick; he was old enough to be her father; and he married her. Probably it was the least caddish thing he ever did. But it was an ill day for Florence.

The April–October romantics lived for a while in Norfolk, Virginia. But Florence's dark angel soon put a stop to that and, through difficulties concerning James Maybrick's business, shuttled them off to a suburb of Liverpool, England, a city where almost anything unpleasant is liable to happen.

The unpleasantness soon set in. James, reverting to Caddishness, started going merrily to hell with the belles and racehorses of Liverpool. And Florence, a young mother though still quite 'unawakened', started herself to toy with the idea of the Primrose Path or, as the Victorians called it, 'going her own way'. It is even reported that she went her own way into a London hotel bedroom with an anonymous gentleman, but at this far date it would be rancorous to cast stones—particularly when one remembers James.

For James was going from bad to worse and from worse to worst. Eventually he reached a peak of Victorian depravity from which there was no going back and little going forward. He took to drugs. Not exclusively, however, to the conventional cocaine or the hackneyed hashish. James was too exotic for that. He favoured the heavy metals. And his pet pick-me-up was arsenic. With increasing frequency he began to patronize the Liverpool chemist shop of a Mr James Heaton where he would replenish his stock of *liquor arsenicalis*—an arsenic solution which he imbibed sometimes as often as five times a day. He found it just the thing for that morning-after queasiness.

Oddly enough, while Mr Maybrick was guzzling arsenic to repair the ravages of his dissipations, Florence had decided that arsenic was just what she needed as a skin lotion to repair the facial ravages caused by her unhappy married life. To obtain this unusual cosmetic, she is reputed to have soaked arsenic out of fly-papers (the old-fashioned sort), a rather messy procedure at which she was unfortunately observed by one of the maids, a certain Alice Yapp, who eventually became as loquacious on the

subject as her name might indicate. Why Mrs Maybrick needed to
endure the sufferings of soaking fly-papers *pour être belle* is a mystery,
since at a later date enough professionally prepared arsenic was found in
the house to poison a whole Panzer Division.

The Maybricks were distinctly an arsenic-conscious family.

In May 1889, James, a gay dog to the end, went to the Wirrall Races,
got wet and returned home next morning feeling very sick in the
stomach. For religious reasons and for the sake of the two young
children, the Maybricks had manfully tried to gloss over the shortcom-
ings of their marriage and were still living in technical harmony. James
was put to bed, visited by a doctor and, in due course, provided with a
day nurse and a night nurse, Nurse Gore and Nurse Callery. Florence,
however, guided by a stern sense of duty, was not willing to leave her
ailing husband to the care of strangers. She herself was a frequent visitor
to the sickroom. According to the nurses, she was too frequent a visitor.
While James went on feeling sicker and sicker in the stomach, she would
try to tempt him with little delicacies of her own contriving, much to the
disgust of the dietetic Nurse Callery. Also she developed a nervous habit
of shuffling bottles and medicaments around on the patient's bed-table.
Her sickroom manner was later described as 'both suspicious and
surreptitious'. And she does seem to have behaved in a rather silly
fashion. One of the silliest things she seemed to have done was to bring
together a bottle of Valentine's Meat Juice and a pinch of some white
powder, believed by many to have been arsenic.

It is hardly startling that, in spite of the ministrations of Nurse Gore
and Nurse Callery, in spite of his wife's tender solicitude, James
Maybrick did not improve. On the 11th of May 1889, he finally passed
away.

Since he had shown symptoms suggesting irritant poisoning, offi-
cious busybodies insisted upon an autopsy, and arsenic was found—not
surprisingly, perhaps—in his body. Actually, the amount discovered was
merely one tenth of a grain, a dose not sufficient to kill a normal
respectable citizen, let alone James. But people feeling the way they do
about arsenic in stomachs, Mrs Maybrick was arrested and charged with
the murder of her husband. Immediately all the silly things she had done
around the bedside came to light. Alice Yapp remembered the fly-
papers. And, before long, the anonymous gentleman and the London
hotel bedrooms were dusted off too.

Florence's bad luck again.

To make matters worse—a sorry fact due, perhaps, less to bad luck than bad management—Mrs Maybrick began to discover that nobody liked her. Her husband's two brothers had never been able to abide her. Now they acted in a most high-handed and spiteful manner, whisking off her children and branding her even before she was accused. Also, Alice Yapp, her fellow servant, Mrs Briggs, Nurse Gore, and Nurse Callery showed the most unfriendly symptoms. They had nothing to say in Mrs Maybrick's favour and seemed to take savage delight in bringing out evidence to her discredit.

Later, when she was brought to trial, the English public didn't like her either. There was something about her.

Perhaps her American blood had a little to do with it. In the Golden Jubilee years of Victoria, American women were frowned upon in England. And the Queen consistently snubbed them when they came to Court. Perhaps they dressed better, looked smarter, and managed to be more amusing than their stolider English sisters. Even the most impeccable Victorian male was not above rolling an appreciative eye at them, so long as they stayed out of trouble. But once they were in the soup, the men were as ready as the women to trace the scarlet 'A' blazing forth beneath the chic American camisoles.

As if this weren't bad luck enough, Mrs Maybrick had bad luck with her jury and terrible luck with one aspect of her defence.

The jury, consisting mostly of simple-natured men, were not the type accustomed to think for themselves on nice points of law. Their professions, perhaps, speak for them. They were three plumbers (three of them!) two farmers, one milliner, one wood-turner, one provision dealer, one grocer, one ironmonger, one house-painter (at that time no ominous trade), and one baker.

In preparing her defence against this literal-minded group of her peers, Mrs Maybrick was advised not to bring forward any evidence as to the true character, the immorality, the dissipation, the general caddishness of her husband. Sentimentalists have held this as a virtue in Florence Maybrick that she adhered so rigidly to the principles of *de mortuis nil nisi bonum.* Actually, it was the smart, but not smart enough, idea of her solicitors that the less James was discredited, the less apparent motive there would seem for his wife's having wanted to murder him.

In consequence of this blunder in psychology, Mrs Maybrick faced trial as an American hussy who had mistreated and deceived a perfectly good English husband, a man, as far as the jury knew, without a blemish on his character. To add to her troubles, her star witness, Mr James Heaton, the chemist from whom Mr Maybrick had so constantly purchased his swig of *liquor arsenicalis*, was so sick when he came to court that his vital evidence was all but inaudible. Even the brilliant rhetoric of her attorney, Charles Russell, later Lord Chief Justice Russell, could not soar above these obstacles.

And, as a final disaster, Mrs Maybrick was not merely facing trial, she was facing Mr Justice Stephen on the bench. In the light of his future career, which ended one year later in the madhouse, Mr Justice Stephen was a little more than even the most callous of murderesses deserved. This once illustrious personage was already losing grip on his sanity before the trial started; all he needed to complete the process was Florence Maybrick. From the beginning he liked her no better than anyone else had. As the trial limped along with no one exactly knowing who did what, his dislike for her swelled within him until it reached almost psychopathic proportion. This manifested itself finally, in his summing-up, as a two-day harangue of impassioned malignity and misogyny. In one of the most biased speeches ever to come from the English bench, he referred to poor Mrs Maybrick as 'that horrible woman' and branded her as the epitome of all that was vile. Startling even the prosecution, he vindictively manœuvred the Valentine's Meat Juice and a certain bottle of glycerine around until he left no loophole for the unlucky woman's innocence.

As obedient Britons, the jury did not hesitate in following the guidance of a Social Superior. As a man, the three plumbers, the two farmers, the milliner, the wood-turner, the grocer, the ironmonger, the house-painter, and the baker brought in a verdict of guilty. Judge Stephen—with a certain rather lunatic satisfaction, perhaps?—donned the black cap and pronounced that Florence Maybrick should be hanged by the neck until she was dead.

A short time later he was himself pronounced insane.

The verdict, coming after a trial in which nothing seemed to have been proved one way or the other, staggered England. It staggered the world. In a few weeks hundreds of thousands of people had signed petitions for Mrs Maybrick's reprieve. Public opinion, in the face of what seemed like gross injustice, swung around to her side. Florence was popular at last.

For two or three weeks she lived (to use her own ill phrase) 'in the shadow of the gallows'. Finally, a little intimidated perhaps by the general clamour, Mr Matthews, the Home Secretary—for there was no Supreme Court of Criminal Appeal at that time—retried the case *in camera* and commuted Mrs Maybrick's sentence to one of penal servitude of life. His reaons for this clemency were that:

> 'Inasmuch as, although the evidence leads to the conclusion that the prisoner administered and attempted to administer arsenic to her husband with intent to murder him, yet it does not wholly exclude a reasonable doubt whether his (James Maybrick's) death was in fact caused by the administration of arsenic.'

In other words, Mr Matthews was of the opinion that Mrs Maybrick had been guilty of attempting to kill her husband with arsenic although it wasn't certain that he had died from arsenical poisoning. This charge was something Mrs Maybrick had not even been tried for during a court procedure at which nothing had been proved beyond the fact that James was dead—a sad eventuality which had been common knowledge before ever the slow-moving wheels of the law had got under way. If that wasn't bad luck—what is?

Whether or not Mrs Maybrick was guilty, and of how much, is no longer calculable. That she was grievously wronged is beyond doubt. The English Bench has never been noted for its chivalry or its leniency towards women accused of murder, particularly where there is also a whiff of adultery. Mrs Thompson, of the haunting love-letters, and other sisters in misfortune reached the gallows as adulteresses rather than murderesses. Mrs Rattenbury alone, that poor darling with her fatal attachment to the boy chauffeur, had a fair deal in this respect. But prudish public opinion soon snuffed her out as efficiently as the hangman's rope.

If Mrs Maybrick learned one thing from her dismal experience, it was that virtue pays dividends when a lady happens to get mixed up in an English murder trial.

That London hotel bedroom turned out to be very expensive.

Mrs Maybrick proceeded from one squalid penal institution to another, suffering all the hardships of a habitual and vicious criminal; conspicuous among which was a period of nine months' solitary confinement. But though her memory had been rinsed off the disdainful hands of British justice, she was not forgotten. Soon a tornado broke from the other side of the Atlantic. American Woman was just beginning to realize herself as a Cosmic Force in 1890. American journalism was making itself felt in Europe. And American public opinion was begining to mean something.

Petitions thick as fleas started to pester various, successive Home Secretaries. In England, Lord Russell himself was active on her behalf, stalwartly proclaiming her innocence. From the American side, Presidents, ambassadors, and their wives, notables in all walks of life, signed formidable statements, one of which, penned by no less a figure than the Honourable James G. Blaine, is worthy of quotation since, with magnificent daring, it snatches the garland of 'snobisme' from its traditional resting-place on the coroneted British heads and hurls it back like a boomerang across the Atlantic. Mrs Maybrick, writes James G. Blaine, was guilty of no crime other than that:

> 'she may have been influenced by the foolish ambition of too many American girls for a foreign marriage, and have descended from her own rank to that of her husband's family, which seems to have been somewhat vulgar. . . .'

This blast at the Maybricks' social position was paralleled in the *North American Review* by the famous American newspaperwoman 'Gail Hamilton', who addressed an open letter to Queen Victoria protesting Mrs Maybrick's innocence, inveighing against her unfair treatment, and begging for her release. But Gail Hamilton and the Honourable James G. Blaine received like treatment. The Queen was neither amused nor interested.

Finally, however, one Home Secretary, Lord Salisbury, goaded beyond endurance by these transatlantic stabs at British justice, parried with a nettled and emphatic statement which might have been penned by the Queen herself. It read in part:

> 'Taking the most lenient view . . . the case of this convict was that of an adulteress attempting to poison her husband under the most cruel circumstances while she was pretending to be nursing him on his sick bed. The Secretary of State regrets that he has been unable to find any grounds for recommending to the Queen any further act of clemency towards the prisoner. . . .'

The women of America continued their losing battle with the stubborn little woman who ruled England. Mrs Maybrick's mother, the Baroness von Roques, is reputed to have spent a fortune in an attempt to have her daughter freed.

All to no purpose, however. Florence served out her sentence, penal servitude for life usually being taken to mean twenty years with three months off a year for good behaviour.

She was finally released in July 1904. On 23 August, shaking the dust of England off her skirts forever, she arrived in New York.

Life held little for her. Both her children, whom she had not seen since the day of her husband's death, had died themselves. Her mother died penniless shortly afterwards. In sore need of money, Florence Maybrick wrote a book—*Mrs Maybrick's Own Story*, published by Funk and Wagnalls in 1905. In this she sang a dismal ballad of atrocities in English gaols and amassed formidable evidence of her own innocence. It is a lugubrious work, filled with lamentable clichés, and poignantly trying to arouse interest in something which once had been a headache but was now only a bore. People read it for its possible sensationalism. They were no longer interested in Mrs Maybrick's misfortunes *per se*. For a while she tried to lecture, largely about conditions in English prisons, but it did not go so well. After a while she began to realize (as Lizzie Borden, settled with her squirrels at 'Maplecroft', had already realized for many years) that people do not take kindly to women who have faced a capital charge, even if they have been shockingly wronged.

Poor Florence! They were back not liking her again.

For several years, in Florida and Highland Park, Illinois, she stubbornly retained her married and now infamous name. But about twenty years before her death she gave up an unequal struggle. Destroying all records of her past and reverting to her maiden name of Florence Chandler, she withdrew to a life of virtual solitude in the tiny three-room shack she had built for herself in the Berkshire Foothills.

There, unknown to her neighbours, she lived on, accepted by the community and, with the years, acquiring from successive generations of South Kent boys the harmless nicknames of 'Lady Florence' and 'The Cat Woman'.

South Kent and Gaylordsville have none but kindly memories of her. There were rumours, at times, of course, as there must be about any lonely little old lady who lives a secluded life, rumours that someone had left her a vast fortune; that a lawyer in a limousine with a liveried chauffeur appeared at regular intervals to bring her cheques. But these were rumours without malice and, unhappily, without foundation in fact, for she died penniless save for an old-age pension finally wooed out of the Government.

South Kent and Gaylordsvill remember her as the little scurrying woman with the walnut face, the gunny-sack, and one loyal and indestructible brown straw hat. To them she was eccentric, yes. It was eccentric in her that she would let no one enter her house; that at night there was always a single light twinkling from her window till morning— to exorcise what demons?—and that with age she had let slip in her squalid little home the niceties of hygiene. But to her neighbours, Mrs Chandler's eccentricities bore no sinister stamp. It was cute rather than grotesque when, fighting against the loss of one of her few remaining teeth, she tied it to its nearest partner with a piece of string. She did no harm, except perhaps to leave a little too many scraps in the wrong places for the campus cats. The South Kent boys liked her.

And they never knew, until the day she died, that the woman they were liking was that most magnificently unliked of women—Mrs Florence Maybrick.

Which leads to the only really comforting feature of this long and uncomfortable life. There in the little village of South Kent and Gaylordsville, Mrs Florence Maybrick found good luck at last—good luck of so sensational a nature that in a way perhaps it neutralized all the tough breaks she had endured earlier.

Mrs Maybrick was able to spend the last twenty years of her life unpersecuted. And yet, had things gone other than the way they did, this lengthy stretch of tranquillity might never have been granted her.

Shortly after her arrival, a neighbour, a Mrs Austin, was kind to Mrs Maybrick and, to show her gratitude, Mrs Maybrick gave her a dress which was trimmed with really good lace. It was undoubtedly the dress in the famous 'wedding' photograph, and to the cynical will perhaps give further proof that there is a real affinity between old lace and arsenic.

When Mrs Austin shook the padding which stuffed the shoulders of this dress, there dropped out a cleaner's card reading: *Mrs Florence Maybrick, Highland Park, Ill.* The name struck a chord in Mrs Austin's memory. She consulted a sister, who in turn consulted a female probation officer in the district. Before long these three women and the two married ladies' husbands knew all the unhappy tale of Mrs Florence Maybrick. A family council was called; the evidence was weighed: and it was decided that she had suffered more than enough already. The Austins and their in-laws thereupon made a vow never to show by word or hint that they knew the real identity of the new arrival.

And so, from the start, 'Mrs Chandler's' future was in the hands of this small group of people. Miraculously, those people kept their vow for twenty years. Never once, at church socials, at whist drives or quilting parties, or at the grocery store, did one of those three ladies succumb to the almost irrestible temptation of launching the juiciest piece of gossip in ten counties.

More power to these gallant ladies of Gaylordsville, so very, very different in character from Alice Yapp, Mrs Briggs, Nurse Gore, and Nurse Callery! More power to these gallant ladies of Gaylordsville who refrained from giving a bad name to a forlorn stray who once had been almost hanged for it!

This was the astounding piece of good luck which came at last and enabled Mrs Maybrick to reach the grave, unwept, perhaps, unhonoured, but at least—unstoned.

On Saturday, 25 October 1941, 'Mrs Chandler' was soberly buried on the South Kent Campus. It had been her own request. Five of the students, boys of 'good stock'—shades of Florence's own beginnings!—were her pall-bearers. These boys, whom a local newspaper with misprinted enthusiasm termed 'Socia*lists* from the swank South Kent School', carried her to her last resting-place. And there, as if a final hand from the grave beckoned her back to respectability, her coffin lies next to that of Miss Doylan, an old friend and beloved South Kent House-mother.

R.I.P. Mrs Florence Chandler Maybrick.

And good luck to you—wherever you are!

CHARLES FRANKLIN
Adelaide Bartlett

Throughout the snowy winter of 1886, England had been agog with the fantastic story of the Pimlico poisoning mystery. The Home Rule Bill, the fall of the Government, riots in the West End and in Belfast, cries in the Balkans and in the Empire, were of relatively minor interest compared with the fascinating Adelaide Bartlett and her strange husband, Edwin, whom she was alleged to have poisoned in the most remarkable and unprecedented manner in the early hours of New Year's Day.

Adelaide Bartlett was one of four very interesting women, each of whom has left an abiding question mark upon the gaslit scene of Victorian Britain. The other three, Madeleine Smith (1857), Florence Bravo (1876) and Florence Maybrick (1889) were each the centre of a lurid *cause célèbre*, after which the question of their guilt remained undecided.

Adelaide Bartlett's acquittal was certainly a controversial one. Everything in fact about the case was sensational and outrageous. It was like a piece of exotic fiction. If a novelist had written it he would have been accused of stretching credibility too far.

The origins of Adelaide Bartlett have always been obscure, as mysterious indeed as the heroine of a Gothic novel. The world had it on the authority of Sir Edward Clarke, Q.C., the man to whose brilliant defence at the Old Bailey Adelaide owed her life, that she was the illegitimate daughter of an Englishman of good family and fortune who had had an affair with an unknown Frenchwoman. She was born at Orléans in 1855 and was christened with the enchanting name of Adelaide Blanche de la Tremouille. She came to England at an early age and was introduced to Edwin Bartlett as his prospective bride when she was an attractive and graceful girl of nineteen. Her father, who refused to own her, bestowed upon her a dowry which, though modest, was greatly welcomed by Bartlett.

Edward Clarke may or may not have got this story from Adelaide herself who was no stickler for the truth. On her marriage certificate her father's name was given as Adolphe Collot de la Tremouille, Comte de Thouars d'Escury, a name which rolls straight out of the Gallic top drawer. It was at one time suggested that Adelaide was fathered by a member of Queen Victoria's entourage during the state visit to Napoleon III in August, 1855. But as Adelaide was born on 20 December, 1855, Her Britannic Majesty's visit can hardly be held responsible for her parentage. The most recent investigations seem to establish that her father's correct name was given on the marriage certificate, and that her mother was an obscure English girl named Clara Chamberlain. It is likely that Adelaide herself was not properly informed about her parentage.

She spent her childhood in France, and was then sent to England to stay with her mother's relatives. Her destiny was controlled by others, and she was always well provided with money. She took to accepting her life thus.

Illegitimacy was a matter for deep shame and disgrace in the nineteenth century. Ordinarily social life was difficult if not impossible for such outcasts. The stain, however, was considerably lightened if one's erring parent was an aristocrat, and particularly an English aristocrat, so great was the awe and reverence in which the upper classes were held. The English milords of the day were gods and their right to seduce girls of the lower classes was barely questioned in a society steeped in puritanical hypocrisy. It was merely necessary to keep it as quiet as possible. Adelaide may well have fancied her father was an English lord. She had a ladylike grace and charm, and her origins were shrouded with the requisite mystery of absentee aristocracy.

At any event, 1875 found her at Kingston-upon-Thames staying with her maternal aunt and uncle, Mr and Mrs William Chamberlain. Among the Chamberlains' friends was Charles Bartlett who ran a removers' business in the town. One day Charles's brother, Edwin, came to visit him. Charles took him to the Chamberlains where Edwin instantly fell in love with Adelaide and wanted to marry her. She was an exceptionally attractive girl. Her dark, fascinating eyes were vibrant with expression. She had a full, beautiful mouth and a lovely complexion, an asset beyond price in the day when ladies were not supposed to use make-up.

Edwin was a prosperous grocer and provision dealer in partnership with Edward Baxter. He was about thirty years old. The marriage was quickly arranged. Adelaide's parents in Orléans, after making judicious inquiries concerning the prospective groom, gave their approval and the modest dowry. The marriage was arranged in typical French style. Afterwards, Adelaide herself said: 'My consent to my marriage was not asked, and I only saw my husband once before my wedding day.'

But the marriage was by no means an unhappy one. Adelaide was a charming and pliable girl, full of natural affection and anxious in every way to please her husband. Edwin, though a man of very strange ideas loved her and was extremely loyal to her. As he was of lowly parentage and had had little education himself, he felt a deep respect for learning and was greatly impressed by Adelaide's aristocratic origins, even if they were on the wrong side of the blanket.

Adelaide, however, had been only sketchily educated a fact of which Edwin was well aware and which he intended to remedy immediately. And so, instead of a honeymoon or, indeed, any kind of married life, he sent her off to a boarding school at Stoke Newington where she remained for two years, living with her husband only during the holidays. After that she went to a finishing school in Belgium. Adelaide submitted unquestioningly to this extraordinary beginning to her married life. The acquisition of learning and the accomplishments of finishing schools were greatly prized in those days and Adelaide may well have been pleased at the opportunity of filling the gaps in her education.

In 1878, her schooling completed, she went to live with her husband in the rooms above one of his shops in Station Road, Herne Hill. He had, very properly he considered, withheld the sexual side of married life from his schoolgirl wife. Edwin was either remarkably abstemious or slightly queer or, as some believed, he was having it off with the ladies of the town. Victorian London, according to the careful investigations of Henry Mayhew, contained 80,000 prostitutes. Brothels to suit all tastes, perversions and pockets abounded. Victorian sex life was lurid and to a large extent the result of the moralists' teaching that the enjoyment of sex was sinful.

Except for one celebrated occasion, the married life of Adelaide and Edwin apparently remained platonic. This at least was the general belief, fostered by Adelaide herself. Edwin treated Adelaide as though she was a piece of Dresden china. He was excessively proud of her and took great delight in showing her off to his friends who were, however, rather few. Adelaide was lonely. Her husband's time was wholly taken up by his business, now greatly enlarged and prospering mainly as the result of his wife's dowry which had been carefully invested in it. He bought Adelaide a couple of dogs upon which she lavished her pent-up affections.

The shadow in her life was her father-in-law and he was to remain so right to the end. Edwin Bartlett senior was a crafty old man whose animosity played a vital part in the tragic story of his son and Adelaide. He was antagonistic to Adelaide right from the start. To begin with, she was French and he disliked all foreigners, particularly the hated French. Secondly she came between him and his son, off whom he had been sponging for some years.

At the time Adelaide went to live at Station Road, Barlett *père* had become a widower and moved in with Edwin and his wife. The old man returned his son's abundant hospitality by being as unpleasant to Adelaide as he could. In 1878 he accused her of having an affair with his youngest son, Frederick.

This brought matters to a head. There was a great scene during which Edwin took his wife's part so strongly that he threatened to throw his father out unless he made a statement before a solicitor retracting his allegations against Adelaide. The old man complied, though with mental reservations, for he had no desire to quarrel with the son who provided him so munificently with the comforts of life. Bartlett senior remained on good terms with his son, visiting him at his places of business almost daily right to the end; but the quarrel with Adelaide was only mended on the surface. They continued to dislike each other as much as ever.

Adelaide Bartlett's sex life has become a matter of considerable importance in the annals of crime. On the surface, it would appear that in Edwin's eyes she stood high on her pedestal, and was too much of a lady to submit to the horrid indignity of physical sex. But there came a time when Adelaide, a warm affectionate creature, found herself very naturally wanting to have a child. That this could not be accomplished without the preliminary of copulation became obvious to her, after she had read a certain book she found in Edwin's library. It was eloquently entitled: *Esoteric Anthropology (The Mysteries of Man): A Comprehensive and Confidential Treatise on the Structure, Functions, Passionate Attractions and Perversions, True and False, Physical and Social Conditions and the Most intimate Relations of Men and Women by* T.L. Nichols, M.D., F.A.S.

It is difficult to believe that a man who wished to protect his wife from the realities of sex should have put this book in her way. Such scandalous reading in a middle-class Victorian household was very unusual. That Adelaide read the book from cover to cover indicates a broadmindedness out of tune with her age, and has led some to believe that it was she who acquired the book herself in the first place, not Edwin.

She learned one vital thing from it: the precise moment in her lunar cycle in which copulation would most likely lead to pregnancy; and according to the Bartlett legend there was one Sunday afternoon, prudently chosen by Adelaide in conjunction with the knowledge she had acquired from Dr Nichols, during which she and Edwin were said to have had their one act of sex in their married life. It duly resulted in her pregnancy.

Certainly a married couple who copulated only once during their married life are deserving of some note. In the case of George IV and Caroline of Brunswick it seems likely enough. But as far as the Bartletts are concerned there is room for doubt; we have it only from Adelaide and her word was not always reliable. Indeed, the legend that Adelaide had fostered about her almost virginal marriage was later upset by Nurse Annie Walker who had the confidence of both Adelaide and Edwin. According to her, the Bartletts always slept together in the same bed; what 'the single act' meant was that they took precautions during sexual intercourse except on that one occasion which led to Adelaide's pregnancy. (A pocket full of french letters found in Edwin's clothes after his death seemed to confirm these statements.)

Nurse Annie Walker, a fully qualified midwife, was installed at Station Road about a month before the baby was due.

Edwin intended to take no chances with his precious wife during this difficult time. Annie Walker had been engaged through the good offices of Mrs Nichols, the wife of the author who had written the *Esoteric Anthropology*. She soon saw that Adelaide was going to have a difficult time, so she suggested to Edwin that a doctor should be called in.

Edwin was dead against this. He didn't want to have 'any man interfering with her'. Nurse Walker told him that it was the baby rather then the mother's life which would be in danger. Adelaide's confinement was so difficult and painful that a doctor was called in at the last minute, but he was too late to save the child. It was born dead.

Annie Walker stayed on for three more weeks until Adelaide was fully recovered. The two women became firm friends. Even after the nurse's professional services were no longer required, she used to visit the Bartletts staying, on at least one occasion, for several days.

She was on extremely friendly terms with both Adelaide and Edwin and was the recipient of many confidences, some of them on the most intimate subjects. Annie Walker later gave evidence at Adelaide's trial, and she said that she found the Bartletts a united and affectionate couple. Adelaide, however, did complain to her about the terms of her husband's will in which he had left everything to her, but only on condition that she did not remarry. In view of what happened later, an ominous interpretation was placed upon this; Adelaide has even been accused of forging the later will which removed the condition. However, she certainly had reason to complain about her husband's first will as his prosperity had been largely brought about by the infusion of her own dowry into his business.

In 1883 they left Station Road and went to live over another of Bartlett's shops in Lordship Lane, East Dulwich. There was no room for Bartlett senior. Much to Adelaide's relief the old man had to find lodgings of his own. He had no financial worries, however. His generous son saw to that.

It was in Lordship Lane that they met Mr and Mrs Matthews. Alice Matthews became an intimate friend of Adelaide's and remained so until her trial. George Matthews was a business associate of Edwin's and the two men also became close friends.

Then, in 1885, when the Bartletts had moved to Merton Abbey, near Wimbledon there was the fatal meeting with the Rev George Dyson. Dyson, a graduate of Trinity College, Dublin, was the minister of the local Wesleyan chapel. He was about twenty-seven years old, had a heavy black moustache and closely trimmed whiskers and was not a man of either striking appearance of personality. He is said to have had dog-like eyes and a permanently wounded expression.

Dyson paid a duty call on the Bartletts. What impressed Edwin more than anything was the fact that the clergyman was a man of education, a university graduate. Edwin hoped that by encouraging the friendship he would be able to bask in culture. The Rev. Dyson's accomplishments in this direction were, as a matter of fact, slight. He was struggling along on a hundred pounds a year, and was envious of the Bartletts' opulence. The real attraction, however, was Mrs Bartlett, with her poise and fascinating accent. The three of them soon became fast friends and Dyson foolishly plunged headlong into a highly dangerous situation, one in which a clergyman should never find himself, for it was soon obvious to him that Edwin was more or less thrusting Adelaide into his arms and encouraging them to be together as much as possible.

It is not an unknown eccentricity for a man to thrust his wife into another man's arms. Watching one's wife being made love to and even copulating with someone else, is a form of masochism well-known to the sexologist. Edwin Bartlett was a strange man with strange ideas. Everyone who knew him said that. One of his favourite theories was that a man should have two wives, one for intelligent companionship and one for domestic purposes, and by the way he behaved over George Dyson, he gave the impression that a wife should have similar privileges.

Instead of being shocked at such un-Victorian notions, the Rev Dyson pursued his intimacy with Edwin and his attractive wife unremittingly. There is little doubt that he became completely fascinated by Adelaide, but his friendship for Edwin remained strong right to the end. Edwin encouraged them to go out for walks together, and to kiss each other in his presence. They were soon kissing each other in secret, though no one knows how far their love-making went, or whether Adelaide became his mistress.

Edwin's remarkable attitude towards Adelaide's relationship with George Dyson was expression in a letter written to him in September, 1885, when the Bartletts were spending a month at Dover. By then the three of them were on Christian name terms.

14 St James Street,
Dover, Monday.

Dear George—Permit me to say I feel great pleasure in thus addressing you for the first time. To me it is a privilege to think that I am allowed to feel towards you as a brother, and I hope our friendship may ripen as time goes on, without anything to mar its future brightness. Would that I could find words to express my thankfulness to you for the very loving letter you sent Adelaide today. It would have done anybody good to see her overflowing with joy as she read it to me. I felt my heart going out to you. I long to tell you how proud I feel at the thought I should soon be able to clasp the hand of the man who from his heart could pen such noble thoughts. Who can help loving you? I felt I must say two words: 'Thank you', and my desire to do so is my excuse for troubling you with this. Looking towards the future with joyfulness, I am yours affectionately,

Edwin.

The Freudian interpretation of this extraordinary letter might be that Edwin was a latent homosexual, and it is certainly possible that his curious make-up might have been complicated by such tendencies, and that he might not have been aware of them.

George's reply to Edwin's strange effusion was modestly naïve.

18 Parkfields, Putney,
September 23, 1885

My dear Edwin—Thank you very much for the brotherly letter you sent me yesterday. I am sure I respond from my heart to your wish that our friendship may ripen with the lapse of time, and I do so with confidence, for I feel that our friendship is founded on a firm, abiding basis—trust and esteem. I have from a boy been ever longing for the confidence and trust of others. I have never been so perfectly happy as when in possession of this. It is in this respect, among many others, that you have shown yourself a true friend. You have thanked me, and now I thank you; yet I ought to confess that I read your warm and generous letter with a kind of half fear—a fear lest you should ever be disappointed in me and find me a far more prosy, matter-of-fact creature than you expect. Thank you, moreover, for the telegram; it was very considerate to send it. I am looking forward with much pleasure to next week. Thus far I have been able to stave off any work and trust to be able to keep it clear. Good old Dover! It will ever possess a pleasant memory for me in my mind and a warm place in your heart. With very kind regards, believe me, yours affectionately.

George.

Taking full advantage of the liberal trust and confidence of his affectionate friend Edwin, George spent as much time as he could with Adelaide at the expense of his flock, and while Edwin was busy in London. He and Adelaide walked hand-in-hand along the sea shore. He knew that he was treading a very indiscreet path, though he did not dream that it would lead him to the dock at the Old Bailey.

George Dyson was a weak and selfish man and there is no doubt at all that he was after Adelaide; but as she was the stronger character of the two, she was no wife to be seduced without her full consent. Moreover, it was obvious that she was extremely fond of Edwin and remained loyal to him to the end, so the balance of probabilities is that Dyson didn't get his way with her.

Besides, a more interesting development took Dyson's attention and riveted him even more firmly to the Bartletts. Edwin made a new will, leaving everything unconditionally to Adelaide; and he appointed George co-executor with his solicitor. Not only was he made executor, but Edwin told George that in the likely event of his death, he wished to give Adelaide to him, and there was apparently something like a betrothal between George and Adelaide.

Precisely how this extraordinary arrangement came about, Dyson himself who was thoroughly questioned about it later was a little vague. He said that his conscience began to smite him about his feelings for Adelaide and that he told both her and Edwin that he was getting too fond of her and that it was disturbing his work.

Edwin wouldn't hear of their friendship being discontinued. On the subject of George having Adelaide, Edwin may not have said more than just: 'If anything happens to me, you two may come together.' That would not have been an extraordinary thing to say by a hypochondriac who might have thought he had not very long to live. If Adelaide and George are to be believed, he very definitely bequeathed his wife to his friend, and the fact was taken for granted between them. There was for instance the occasion when Adelaide did or said something which neither man approved, and which drew the comment from George: 'When she comes under my care, I shall have to teach her differently.'

Adelaide went so far as to state specifically that her husband had given her to George Dyson whom she regarded as her fiancé. And according to her own words, she took her 'betrothal' to Dyson very seriously.

In the August of 1885 the Bartletts moved to London and took furnished rooms on the first floor of 85 Claverton Street, Pimlico, the house of Mr and Mrs Frederick Doggett, Mr Doggett, by some strange quirk of irony, was a Registrar of Births and Deaths.

George Dyson swallowing the rising tide of his conscience continued his delicious, if slightly frustrating affair with Adelaide. After all, it was Edwin's most ardent wish. During the last months of his life Edwin continued to enjoy his unhusbandly pleasure of watching Adelaide and George issing each other. He encouraged them to spend days alone together, and to further this end he bought George a season ticket from Putney to Waterloo. George was supposed to be giving Adelaide instruction in such subjects as Latin, history, geography and mathematics.

He stayed with her all day alone in the Claverton Street sitting-room, and his presence aroused considerable comment.

The Doggetts' maid surprised them in affectionate attitudes—on the sofa together, her head on his shoulder, him sitting on a low chair, her on the floor, her head on his knee. Once the maid surprised them on the floor together. The curtains were always pulled and there was never a sign of instruction of any intellectual nature going on.

Dyson's mind must have been simplicity itself. But Adelaide was no fool. It is difficult to know what went on in her mind to permit herself to be a party to this extraordinary affair. Even if she believed Edwin when he said he had not long to live, and if she had agreed that Dyson should have her next, why did she not have the delicacy to await the expected demise? Could she have been persuaded that she was filling Edwin's last months with pleasure by kissing and flirting with George in his presence? That Edwin looked upon her more as his daughter than his wife?

Whatever she thought, it seems that this curious exercise in voyeurism was having the effect of arousing—or rearousing—Edwin's desire for Adelaide which was to have fatal consequences. Adelaide no longer shared his bed. She had insisted on sleeping separately. There was one simple reason. Edwin had for some years suffered greatly with his teeth. A quack dentist had sawn his bad teeth off at gum level and fixed him with a denture which naturally led to endless dental trouble. As a consequence of all this, his breath became extremely foul and offensive, so much so that his fastidious wife could not endure him coming close.

Edward, a hypochondriac, believed that he was suffering from some fearful disease. He was always dosing himself with pills and medicines, and among the things he took was mercury. It was never discovered why he took this particular toxic which was a standard cure for syphilis at the time. (Hence the theory that he had frequented prostitutes rather than soil his immaculate wife.) But although Bartlett actually suffered from the delusion that he had syphilis there was no post-mortem evidence for this disease later on.

Early in December he took to his bed with sickness and diarrhoea. Adelaide tenderly nursed him and summoned Dr Alfred Leach who found him suffering from a pain in his left side, diarrhoea and gastritis. Edwin received several visits from the dentist who removed bad teeth and stumps. This, combined with Dr Leach's treatment, brought about a rapid recovery in Edwin's health. Actually there was nothing much wrong with him, but he remained miserable and depressed. He suffered from delusions, had fits of hysteria and wept by the hour. All the time Adelaide performed the unpleasant tasks of the sick-room willingly and without complaint. Night after night she sat beside his bed on an easy chair, snatching what sleep she could and refusing to go to bed herself.

Edwin's malevolent father paid frequent visits but was admitted to the sick-room only three times by Adelaide who did not want Edwin disturbed by his father's ill-natured suspicions. She told the old man plainly that she had neither forgiven nor forgotten the quarrel at Station Road. She knew well enough that her father-in-law still believed the worst of her, mainly on the grounds that she was a foreigner. The evil-minded old man haunted Claverton Street, muttering vague and menacing accusations.

Although Dr Leach was satisfied with the progress of his patient, Mrs Bartlett suggested they should get another opinion. Edwin himself was firmly against this. He was quite content with Dr Leach's treatment.

But Adelaide insisted upon a second doctor being called in and gave the startling prophetic reason: 'If Mr Bartlett does not get better soon, his friends and relations will accuse me of poisoning him.' Edwin then agreed to the second opinion merely in order to protect Adelaide against his friends and relations, particularly his ill-natured father.

Dr Leach brought in a certain Dr Dudley who found Edwin depressed, complaining of lack of sleep. His gums were 'spongy and inflamed'. Otherwise there was nothing the matter with him. He told him he ought to get up and go out every day.

George Dyson was a constant, sympathetic visitor and there is no reason to think that the feeling between the two men had changed. But according to Adelaide a change came over Edwin about this time. His mental deterioration has already been noted. He became neurotic and hysterical and he suffered from delusions. He also developed a desire to reclaim his right of the marriage bed which to Adelaide was apparently incomprehensible—in view of the fact that she was betrothed to George—and nauseating on account of his fetid breath.

On 27 December Adelaide asked George Dyson to get her a quantity of chloroform privately. She told him that Edwin suffered from some painful internal complaint about which the doctor knew nothing, the spasms of which could only be soothed by the use of chloroform.

Edwin died on the ast day of December. After a meal of half a dozen oysters, he went to have some teeth extracted under gas. Dr Leach and Adelaide accompanied him. In the cab Adelaide mentioned to the doctor that she and her husband were saying only that morning that they wished they were unmarried so that they could have the pleasure of getting married all over again. 'That is very flattering to you, Mr Bartlett,' remarked Leach. Edwin was all muffled up and his reply was inaudible.

The dentist drew Leach's attention to the state of necrosis in Edwin's gums. There is little doubt that Edwin heard the dread word necrosis. He took a long time—four minutes—before he became unconscious by the gas. Otherwise the operation was quickly and successfully performed.

Edwin and Adelaide returned to Claverton Street where there was a conversation with Mrs Doggett on the subject of taking chloroform. Mrs Doggett had had an operation some years previously—was not the sensation of taking chloroform 'nice and pleasant'? asked Adelaide. Mrs Doggett could not really agree that it was. Adelaide said that she was in the habit of administering sleeping drops to her husband.

Edwin, whatever else might have been the matter with him, was not off his food. For dinner he had jugged hare, for supper more oysters and several delicacies including chutney and he ordered a large haddock for breakfast.

Mr and Mrs Doggett had friends in to celebrate the New Year with them. Upstairs Adelaide sat silently beside her husband's bed, listening to the sounds of the New Year celebrations below. At a quarter past midnight the Doggetts went to bed. The house was wrapped in silence until four o'clock in the morning when Adelaide awakened the Doggetts and told them that she thought her husband was dead. She had already sent the maid for Dr Leach.

Leach was completely confounded. He could find no reason for his patient's death. Adelaide said she awoke in her bedside chair to find Edwin lying twisted over on his side, face downwards. She said she had poured brandy down his throat in a vain effort to revive him. On the mantelpiece, within the dead man's reach, was a glass containing liquid, smelling like 'chloric ether'.

'Could he have taken poison?' asked Leach. Adelaide held that to be impossible, as he could not have got poison without her knowledge.

Leach declined to give a death certificate, saying there must be a post-mortem. Adelaide agreed to this and urged him to make the examination as soon as possible.

On the mantelpiece was a bottle of chlorodyne which, Adelaide assured the doctor, Edwin used to rub on his gums. Then he must have swallowed some, suggested Leach. If Adelaide had really murdered her husband, why did she not jump at this explanation which might have prompted the sympathetic Dr Leach, who had always been susceptible to her charms and the magnetism of her dark eyes, to sign the death certificate there and then? Instead, she positively insisted on the post-mortem examination. 'Spare no expense,' she said.

Dr Green, of Charing Cross Hospital, was unable to perform the autopsy until the following day. While Adelaide was distraught and chaffing at the delay, her father-in-law arrived at the house, bristling with suspicion. He kissed his son and ostentatiously smelt his mouth for signs of prussic-acid poisoning.

'We must have a post-mortem,' he said to Leach. 'This cannot pass.' The doctor informed him curtly that it had already been arranged. After looking round for signs of hidden poisons, the old curmudgeon kissed Adelaide goodbye and went off to make as much trouble for her as he possibly could.

The post-mortem took place on 2 January. The doctors were unable to discover any natural cause for death. They took the stomach away for examination.

With suspicions mounting around her—those of her father-in-law being the meanest and most persistent—Adelaide went to stay with her friends, the Matthews.

She kept her dignity and her head. The Rev George Dyson, however, was in a state of panic. Though obviously Adelaide was the one under the deepest suspicion, he had no thought or consideration for anyone but himself. To give her the solace of his Christian office was the last thing in his mind.

As the days passed and the suspense mounted, his behaviour completely altered her feelings towards him. They had rows at the Matthews's house. Dyson found out that chloroform had been found in Edwin's stomach and he naturally enough wanted to know what Adelaide had done with the chloroform he had bought for her.

Adelaide was very angry. 'Oh damn the chloroform!' she exclaimed stamping her foot. Mrs Matthews—doubtless listening at the door—broke in on the scene to hear Dyson say, 'You did tell me that Edwin was going to die soon.' Adelaide denied that she had said anything of the kind. Dyson bowed his head, moaning, 'My God, I am a ruined man.' He warned her that he was determined to make a clean breast of the affair, although Adelaide asked him not to mention the chloroform.

In their more affectionate days Dyson had been in the habit of penning little verses to Adelaide. An example of his poetic powers has been handed down to posterity:

> Who is it that hath burst the door,
> Unclosed the heart that shut before,
> And set her queen-like on her throne,
> And made its homage all her own?
> My Birdie

Dyson now wanted the return of this deathless piece, and his 'Birdie' obliged him with fitting scorn.

On 16 January, she and Dyson had another interview. According to him, she told him that he was distressing himself unnecessarily—if he did not incriminate himself, *she* would not incriminate him.

Their last meeting before they appeared together in the dock at the Old Bailey was three days later at the Matthews's house where, according to him, she told him that she had retrieved the chloroform bottle from Claverton Street, had emptied the contents out of the railway carriage between Victoria and Peckham Rye, and thrown the bottle into a pond.

He said: 'Supposing it should be proved that you——

'Don't mince matters,' she interrupted. 'Why not say I gave him the chloroform?'

Late in January the Home Office analyst found that a quantity of chloroform in the stomach had been the sole cause of Edwin Bartlett's death. When Dr Leach imparted this information to Adelaide expecting it to take a load off her mind, he was surprised to find her strangely agitated.

It was then that she confided in him about her husband's curious ideas of marriage and about the strange triangular relationship between herself, her husband and George Dyson.

During the latter stages of his illness, Adelaide said, Edwin wished to assert his martial rights. She had pointed out to him the impropriety of such conduct. 'Edwin,' she said, 'you have given me to Mr Dyson, and it is not right that you should now do what during all these years of our married life you have not done.' She had protested strongly against Edwin's behaviour, as it was 'a duty which she owed to her womanhood and to the man to whom she was practically affianced'. He apparently agreed with what she said, but when he got better, his desire for her became so urgent that she bought chloroform, intending to sprinkle some on a handkerchief and wave it in front of his face when he became too pressing. She did not, however, attempt to put this plan into action.

She never had any secrets from Edwin, she declared, and the presence of the chloroform in the drawer so troubled her that, on New Year's Eve, she told him all about it. She gave him the bottle when he was in bed. 'He was not angry. He looked at it and placed it on the corner of the mantelpiece close to his bed.' She then went to sleep and awoke to find him dead.

Dr Leach made little comment when he heard the strange story which Adelaide imagined was made in complete confidence. But he assured her that the chloroform would not have had the effect on Edwin which she apparently expected.

The Coroner's inquest was held in February to the accompaniment of enormous public interest. Dr Leach recounted the story of Adelaide Bartlett's remarkable confidences. Medical evidence established that eleven and a quarter grains of alcohol were found in the deceased's stomach. Adelaide, on legal advice, declined to give evidence. But the Rev George Dyson availed himself of the opportunity of 'making a clean breast of things'.

He told the story of the chloroform in detail. He had been deceived and duped by a wicked woman, so he claimed, deliberately thrown into her company by her husband, and as a consequence found himself 'attacked upon his weakest side'. His treachery to Adelaide and the way he tried to put all the blame on her resulted in her immediate arrest at the request of the Coroner's jury, but he failed to save his own reputation, for he was later arrested and charged as being an accessory before the fact. The Coroner's jury returned a verdict of wilful murder against Adelaide.

On 13 April, they both stood side by side in the dock at the Old Bailey before Mr Justice Wills. Dyson was nervous and uneasy and kept stealing glances at the woman with whom he had been so guiltily in love and whom he had so basely betrayed.

But Adelaide, drawn and composed, gazed straight ahead and did not give Dyson one glance. Her appearance in the dock caused something of a sensation. Her widow's weeds were gone and in defiance of the convention of the day she was hatless. Her hair had been cut short and was arranged in a halo of curls around her head. The v-line of her black, tightly-fitting dress was edged with white lace. Slender and poised, she looked pathetically appealing.

As soon as she had come under suspicion of causing the death of her husband, Adelaide's mysterious parent had come to her aid. Unlimited funds were placed at her disposal to provide her with the best legal advice and protection. Edward Clarke, Q.C., M.P., the greatest defence advocate of the day, had been briefed to defend her as early as 20 February, two days after the verdict of the Coroner's jury.

Although Adelaide Bartlett was perhaps the most interesting woman to be charged with murder in nineteenth-century England, the real hero of her trial was Edward Clarke. His defence of her has gone down in history as one of the greatest performances at the English bar.

He had an extremely difficult task. Public opinion was wholly against her. Everyone believed her guilty before the trial began, a state of affairs which naturally affects the minds of a jury. The circumstances of her married life were bizarre and greatly offensive to Victorian ideas. Her own story was not only scandalous, but difficult to believe. The fact that she was of foreign origin did not exactly help her case either.

Clarke was not a man who sought the limelight. He was a great humanitarian and Adelaide Bartlett aroused his deepest sympathy. Here was a woman, hounded by her relatives, abandoned by all her friends, including the Matthews, vilified by public opinion, condemned unheard.

When Adelaide stood in the box at the Old Bailey she had not a single visible friend in the world. The only humanity shown to her had been by the officials at Clerkenwell Prison and by her solicitor who handled her husband's and now her affairs. What she was to owe to Edward Clarke's singleminded devotion to her cause only transpired later.

In those days the defendant was now allowed to go into the witness-box and give evidence. Whether this was a good thing or a bad thing is an interesting legal argument. It is certain that Adelaide would have endured a terrible and agonizing cross-examination from Sir Charles Russell, the Attorney-General and the most deadly cross-examiner of his day, from which she would not have emerged unscathed.

Edward Clarke had the advocate's supreme gift—that of persuasion; and the task he set himself to persuade the jury that Adelaide Barlett's own story was true. He called no evidence himself. All the witnesses appeared for the Crown. Their evidence he brilliantly exploited in cross-examination. He was sometimes highly destructive, but more often and with amazing subtlety he turned the witness's own words to his client's advantage.

Clarke was one of the busiest counsel of the day and was greatly in demand. His desk was piled with lucrative briefs, but he dropped everything to defend Adelaide Bartlett. He spent days in the British Museum library studying the medical effects of chloroform. His whole mind concentrated on nothing but this one case—unlike the Attorney-General who was deeply involved in one of the great political issues of the day and did not bring the full force of his intelligence to bear upon the presentation of the prosecution.

Every day Edward Clarke arrived early in court, so that he was sitting there in his place when the prisoner was brought into the dock, and every day he gave this friendless and lonely woman a smile of encouragement. He knew what that meant to her. It was typical of the humanity of this great advocate. Adelaide was soon to discover what a great and powerful defender she had in court.

The trial began, as it continued and ended, in sensation. As soon as the charges were read, the Crown withdrew the case against George Dyson. He stepped from the dock a free man, and doubtless without a single thought for his former love whom he left alone to face the dread charge of murder.

Edward Clarke smiled encouragingly at the forlorn figure in the dock. He knew—she did not—that Dyson's acquittal could be turned to her advantage, for he would now have to give evidence for the Crown. Clarke wrote later: 'Having admitted that he was innocent, the Attorney-General could not help calling him as a witness, and so offering him for my cross-examination. That would not be hostile, but friendly and sympathetic, for the more closely I could associate his actions with those of Mrs Bartlett, the more I should strengthen the instinctive reluctance of the jury to send her to the hangman's cord, while he passed unrebuked to freedom.'

In his opening speech for the Crown the Attorney-General posed the vital question: How did the chloroform get into Edwin Bartlett's stomach? There were three alternatives, he said. Suicide, though there was nothing to suggest he would take his life. Accident, but no man would drink a liquid giving such agonizing pains without immediately perceiving the mistake he had made. The third alternative was deliberate administration by another person.

His theory was that Adelaide had first chloroformed her husband into insensibility and then poured the liquid chloroform down his throat.

Edwin Bartlett senior took the stand and gave his biased evidence against his daughter-in-law. He had worked hard to get her into the dock, yet his evidence had no real bearing on the prosecution's case. His object was to cover Adelaide with as much suspicion as possible. Calling him at all was not a very wise move on the part of the Crown, and old Bartlett's triumph was short-lived, for Edward Clarke thoroughly discredited him in his subsequent cross-examination.

Clarke soon made old Bartlett admit that he had disliked Adelaide from the start. He raked up the apology which the dead man had forced his father to sign concerning the allegations he had made against Adelaide. The old man admitted in court that even though he had signed the apology, he still believed his calumnies were true. He further admitted that he had entered a caveat against his son's will in order to try to get the money himself. The contemptible old man left the box with barely a shred of his character left.

Clarke dealt entirely differently with the Rev George Dyson who gave evidence on the second day. He could easily have shown Dyson up for the weak, despicable creature he was—a man who was prepared to send the woman he said he loved to the gallows to save his own reputation. It was his statements more than anything which had placed Adelaide in the dock. He gave his evidence in a manner hostile and damaging to her. The temptation to annihilate Dyson, as he had done old Bartlett, must have been great. But Edward Clarke's job was to persuade the jury of Adelaid's innocence, not to destroy the character of the man whose intimate association with her presumed to be the motive for her guilt. By destroying Dyson's character, Clarke would also have destroyed that of his client.

He treated Dyson with kid gloves, perhaps rather to Dyson's surprise, for this curious man must surely have suffered in his conscience over what he was doing to Adelaide.

Skilfully Clarke got a number of valuable admissions out of Dyson. He said that Bartlett was a man of very strange ideas, a fact which Clarke used to support the truth of the extraordinary story which Adelaide had told Dr Leach. Dyson also admitted that Bartlett had believed he suffered from a terrible disease of which he would soon die. Clarke persuaded him to admit that Adelaide had not asked him to keep secret the purchase of the fatal chloroform. Dyson, too, had thrown away the bottles he had bought containing the chloroform, for fear of being associated with Bartlett's death. Adelaide had done the same. If Dyson's motives had not been incriminating—for the Crown had admitted him guiltless—why should similar acts of Adelaide be considered so? Clarke was thus skilfully building up the case for his client's innocence, brick by brick.

Dr Leach recounted the illness and death of Edwin Bartlett and read the notes which he had made at the post-mortem. Leach was a tiresome and self-conscious witness, who qualified almost every answer with uncalled-for explanations. He greatly tried the patience of both Judge and Counsel.

He spoke of the great devotion with which the accused nursed her husband. He explained that Edwin had been in an extremely neurotic state, hysterical, eccentric, unbalanced—so much so that Leach suspected at one time that he was insane. Clarke made much of the fact that Adelaide wanted the post-mortem as soon as possible, and also that the longer it was delayed the less likely was it that the true cause of death could be established.

Clarke finally got some important information out of Leach who had frequently administered chloroform. The effect of what Leach said was that, if Mrs Bartlett had made her husband inhale chloroform in order to render him unconscious, and then poured the liquid down his throat—which was the Crown's contention—then Bartlett would almost certainly have vomited, for he had recently had a large meal which included mango chutney. But no vomiting had taken place.

How then did the liquid chloroform get into his stomach?

The Crown now produced its expert medical witnesses. The chief of these was Dr Thomas Stevenson, Professor of Medical Jurisprudence at Guy's Hospital, London, a toxicologist of international standing. He said he knew of no recorded case of murder by the administration of liquid chloroform. It *was* possible to pour liquid chloroform down the throat of an unconscious person, but Clarke made him admit that it was an extremely ticklish and delicate operation—and one so difficult that he would be afraid of pouring it down the windpipe, should he perform it himself. The post-mortem had established that none of the chloroform had gone down Bartlett's windpipe, for it would have left traces behind if it had.

The Crown's case had closed. Edward Clarke offered no evidence. His defence was a magnificent speech, long remembered as a brilliant example of forensic eloquence and skilfully persuasive advocacy.

Before he dealt with the details of the evidence, he summed up the prosecution's case in devastating fashion.

'It is a marvellous thing that you are asked by the prosecution to accept. You are asked to believe that a woman who for years had lived in friendship and affection with her husband, who during the whole time of his illness had striven to tend him, to nurse him and help him, who had tended him by day, who had sacrificed her own rest to watch over him at night, had spent night after night without going to her restful bed, simply giving to herself sleep at the bottom of his couch that she might be ready by him to comfort him by her presence, who had called doctors, who had taken all the pains that the most tender and affectionate nurse possibly could, that by no possibility should any chance be lost of the doctors' ascertaining what his trouble was, and having the quickest means to cure it; you are asked to imagine that that woman on New Year's Eve was suddenly transformed into a murderess, committing crime not only without excuse, but absolutely without any object; you are asked to believe that by a sort of inspiration she succeeds in committing that crime by the execution of a delicate and difficult operation—an operation which would have been delicate and difficult to the highest trained doctors that this country has in it.'

Dealing with the prosecution's theory that the accused had first made her husband unconscious by inducing him to inhale chloroform, and then pouring it down his throat, he said that the expert evidence showed that an attempt to chloroform a sleeping person would cause him to wake up and resist, and that it was extremely unlikely that an unskilled person would be able to do it.

In similar manner Clarke went into great detail to discredit the other evidence presented against Adelaide. The packed court was hushed, listening avidly to his every word. Barristers crowded the benches to hear him. But no one listened to him more ardently than the slight, pale young woman in the dock, to whom his speech was the most important thing in her life. Clarke concluded in memorable style:

'This woman has not had the happiest of lives. She has been described to you as one who had no friends. But she had one friend— her husband. He did stand by her, strange as his ideas may have been, disordered as it would seem from some things that have been said, his intellect in some respects must have been. Yet in his strange way he stood by her and protected her. He was affectionate in manner, and when her reputation was assailed, he defended it as only the husband could defend it. And to her at this moment it may seem most strange that he to whom she had given this persistent affection, even during the years of such a life, should be the one of whose foul murder she now stands accused. And if he himself could know what passed among us here— how strange, how sorrowful it might seem to him—how strange that such an accusation should have been formulated and tried in court, in spite of the efforts which he endeavoured to make to prevent it—the precautions which perhaps by his own rash despairing act he too defeated.

'Gentlemen, that husband has gone. But she is not left without a friend. She will find that friend here today in the spirit which guides your judgement and clears your eyes upon this case. The spirit of justice is in this court today to comfort and protect her in the hour of her utmost need. It has strengthened, I hope, my voice. It will, I trust, clear your eyes and guide your judgement. It will speak with the evidence which I hope and believe has demolished and destroyed the suspicion which rests on her. And that spirit will speak in firm, unfaltering voice when your verdict tells the whole world that in your judgement Adelaide Bartlett is not guilty.'

Edward Clarke sat down to a thunder of applause which Judge and court officials tried sternly but in vain to quell.

The speech of the Attorney-General, who was not at his best owing to his political involvement, and the Judge's summing-up came as an anti-climax to Edward Clarke's brilliant oration.

Mr Justice Wills was a fanatical puritan. He had a thin, cruel mouth, and smouldering eyes which showed little understanding of his fellow human beings. He was boiling with indignation about the *Esoteric Anthropology*, the book which had enlightened Adelaide on sex matters, and he spent some time fulminating about it, expressing his shock and outrage that such 'garbage', such 'outpouring of impurity' should be permitted to corrupt the minds of the public. Indeed, he seemed more shocked about the book than the alleged murder of its owner.

The Judge believed in Adelaid's guilt, but the jury did not listen to him. The words of Edward Clarke were still in their ears when after two hours they found her not guilty, saying that 'although we think grave suspicion is attached to the prisoner, we do not think there is sufficient evidence to show how or by whom the chloroform was administered'.

Clarke had changed public opinion in favour of Adelaide's innocence, and the verdict was greeted with roars of cheering and applause which the irritated Judge said was an outrage.

Overwhelmed, Edward Clarke broke down and wept while Adelaide passed silently out of the court. A week later she wrote him the following letter:

66 Gresham Street
April 24th

Dear Sir—Forgive me for not earlier expressing my heartfelt gratitude to you. I feel that I owe my life to your earnest efforts, and though I cannot put into words the feelings that fill my heart, *you* will understand all that my pen fails to express to you.

Your kind looks towards me cheered me very much, for I felt that you believed me innocent. I have heard many eloquent Jesuits preach, but I never listened to anything finer than your speach *(sic)*

My story was a very painful one, but sadly true. My consent to my marriage was not asked, and I only saw my husband once before my wedding day

I am much gratified that Dr Stevenson has written to say that he concurs in the verdict, he wrote so kindly of Miss Wood who has been a true friend. I received great kindness at Clerkenwell from the Govenor *(sic)* to the lowest, they did their best to comfort me.

Assuring you that I shall always remember you with feelings of deepest gratitude, I am,

Sincerely yours,
Adelaide Bartlett.

The Miss Wood she referred to was the sister of her solicitor, Mr E.N. Wood, at whose home Adelaide stayed as a guest for several weeks after her acquittal. It has been said that while she was in Clerkewell she enjoyed many privileges. The protecting hand was there all the time to give her help and ease her burden.

But many continued to believe that she was guilty and had got away with it, among them Sir James Paget of St Barts Hospital, Queen Victoria's surgeon, who demanded that now the trial was over 'she should have told us in the interests of science how she did it'. There will always be those who question her innocence. Did she perhaps have some strange power over Edwin? He affirmed that he was able to draw currents of strength from her, and then there was a peculiar conversation with the doctor about mesmerism. Did she at the end persuade him, by some form of hypnotism, to drink the chloroform—overwhelmed perhaps at the prospect of having to endure him for the rest of his life? Some think he was in terror of Adelaide and that she completely dominated him.

Edward Clarke was firmly convinced that Edwin Bartlett had committed suicide, fearful of the dread word necrosis, which he might have thought meant that he had developed gangrene. Dr Leach, writing later in *The Lancet*, thought Edwin took the chloroform 'Out of sheer mischief, with the intention of alarming by his symptoms the wife who an hour or two before had talked about using it in an emergency'.

While the great controversy raged, Adelaide left them to it, stealing away, taking her mystery and her strange charm with her. She went to the obvious place, back to Orléans where she was born. Little of life remained, except Edwin's fortune and the great family who only half recognized her and to whom she had been an acute embarrassment.

The Indestructible Man

He flapped his arms and beat his hands against his sides to stir up the circulation as he shuffled along the streets of New York's Bronx that bitter night in mid-December. He wore no overcoat (he had pawned it to buy whisky a few weeks before), and a savage wind that seemed to come straight from the North Pole pressed his threadbare trousers flat against his legs, and whistled through a hole in the crown of his dilapidated hat. It was a few minutes before 9 o'clock when Michael Malloy turned into clamorous Third Avenue and shambled north to 171st Street, heading for his haven—Tony's speakeasy, up the street a few paces. For this was the Prohibition Era.

Malloy passed through the dismal frosted outer door of the shabby store-front establishment into a cheerless vestibule, and pressed a buzzer. Presently a slot in an inner door slid back and a pair of eyes appeared in the opening, carefully scrutinising the customer.

'What the hell!' rasped the man behind the peephole. 'You here again?'

'Now wait a minute, lad,' chirped Malloy in a voice whose timbre had been greatly altered by years of over-indulgence in alcohol. 'I'll pay you Tuesday if you'll give me just one little one.'

'Aw, all right. Come on in.' The door was unlatched, and Malloy made a beeline across the splintery wooden floor to the bar. The man who had let him in—a tough-looking individual with flaming red hair—grudgingly poured out a jigger of 'smoke,' and shoved it towards Malloy.

The derelict (Malloy had been a piece of human flotsam for well over 10 years) was the only person on the front side of the bar that night. For Tony, despite the fact that he·peddled his smoke at two shots to the quarter dollar, had been hit by the depression.

But there were two men in the back room who were watching with speculative eyes as Malloy downed his drink. They were Tony Marino, 27, the proprietor, a typical spawn of Prohibition, who'd pat you on the back in order to find a spot to plant a knife, and Tony's friend Frankie Pasqua, an undertaker by profession, a drunkard by recreation. Pasqua, too, was on the right side of 30. He wore striped trousers, cutaway coat, and a winged collar. He'd just buried somebody this afternoon, and come straight to Tony's. Despite his sartorial splendour, you still wouldn't have wanted to meet up with Mr Pasqua in a dark alley.

Tony Marino had a way with women. Three years before, he'd met up with a blonde streetwalker named Maybelle Carlson, attractive after a fashion. Maybelle had been a frequenter of the speakeasy. Tony always saw to it that she got all she wanted to drink. Often, when Maybelle had more than she could carry, Tony took her home to a tawdry rooming-house not far from his place.

One day, Maybelle was found dead in her room. The police noted that the young lady had practised the peculiar custom of sleeping nude and uncovered, and with the window wide open, in the dead of winter. A physician ascribed death to pneumonia.

And so Maybelle Carlson was buried, Pasqua officiating in his best graveside manner. Two weeks later, Tony Marino received a cheque from an insurance company for 1,500 dollars. Tony, peculiarly enough, had been named the beneficiary in a policy taken out by Miss Maybelle Carlson some few months prior to her untimely demise . . .

And now, by that bitter night in mid-December of 1932, Pasqua, like Tony, had been struck by the Depression. People were still dying, but the undertaker wasn't getting as much for putting them away. And people were drinking as much as ever, Tony told him, but he wasn't getting as much for the stuff.

'Well, who the hell's got all the money, anyway?' the undertaker asked.

Tony made no reply, but sat there, brooding. No money, few customers, fewer friends. Then he suddenly looked up, an evil light in his dark eyes.

'I got an idea, Frankie,' he said. 'If you get a guy I can take insurance out on, I'll give you the undertaking job.'

The words were no sooner out of Tony's mouth than Michael Malloy entered.

'How about him?' The undertaker tilted his head ever so slightly.

Tony followed Pasqua's gaze, and his eyes found Malloy. Malloy, who had spent half of his 40 years in a state of almost continual intoxication. Malloy, this jobless bum who came in with a quarter at the most, then hung around the place all night, wheedling drinks out of the others.

'An idea,' answered Tony. 'An idea.'

Out in the bar, Malloy was negotiating for another drink and Red, the bartender—right name Daniel Murphy—was hurling verbal aspersions on Malloy's parentage.

In the back room, Tony snapped his fingers, and Red came hustling in.

'Give 'im anything he wants,' Tony told Red.

The baretender's eyebrows lifted.

'Don't stand there! Give 'im anything he wants, I tell you!' snapped Tony.

Red went back to the bar to pour Malloy another drink.

Malloy left around midnight, staggering out into a sleet storm, and Tony had the place closed up and the lights put out. Then he called Red into the back room.

It was there, as those three men sat huddled over a cheap table, as the sleet pelted against the windowpanes out in front, that the 'murder trust' was formed.

Michael Malloy was to be murdered—murdered for insurance. Tony would take out the insurance. Red was instructed to give Malloy anything he wanted—and more. Red was further told to buy a gallon of anti-freeze mixture—composed largely of wood alcohol—for the special benefit of Mr Malloy.

The plot included giving Malloy a few rounds of the usual stuff, then switching to the poison. Marino would arrange for the death certificate. And Frankie Pasqua would be in attendance at the requiem and officiate at the grave.

Red ventured the question as to why Malloy had been chosen.

'Because,' said Tony, 'he ain't got no relations.'

The whisk-whisk of Red's broom was all that could be heard for the next hour as the two arch-plotters talked in low, ominous tones, perfecting the final details of what was to turn out to be an epic of horror.

A few nights later, Michael Malloy pressed the buzzer in the vestibule. A slot slid open and a pair of eyes peered through.

'Oh, hello, Malloy. Come on in!'

Malloy's head jerked up a bit. Instead of being threatened with the bum's rush, he was being received with open arms. But Malloy didn't stop to wonder why. It was cold outside again tonight, and a few shots of Tony's stuff would warm him up no end.

Tony, that very morning, had succeeded in obtaining a 1,200-dollar policy on Malloy's life, paying the first quarterly premium in advance, so that the policy went into immediate effect. The insurance salesman, in his keenness to collect his commission, had permitted Tony to sign Malloy's name to the application.

Malloy followed his usual course to the bar—the shortest distance between the door and the nearest part of the brass rail.

'A shot of the same,' he said to Red.

'Sure thing, Malloy. Anything you want,' answered Red. 'And pay whenever you feel like it.'

After half a dozen jiggers of Tony's smoke, Michael Malloy was beginning to feel a little better.

Red, who had looked into the back room after he served each drink, saw Tony give him the nod.

'Have another, Malloy?' asked Red.

'Don't care if I do' Malloy banged his glass down on the bar, and Red picked it up. This time, the bartender poured Malloy a straight shot of anti-freeze mixture. Then, he, Tony and the undertaker in the back room looked on as the derelict lifted the glass of poison to his lips.

Malloy's right hand went through that quick upward jerk of the drunkard, and the glass was empty.

The three plotters knew it would be but a minute or two before Malloy would keel over in his tracks, dead.

A minute passed. Then two. Malloy began to look around the place. It seemed to Tony and the undertaker that he was staring straight at them. They moved a little in their chairs, so that the green curtain separating the bar and the back room would prevent Malloy seeing him.

Then their victim shifted his gaze to the bartender. Tough as he was, Red winced involuntarily, knowing what he had done.

'Now look here, my lad,' Malloy said, a trace of anger in his voice, 'you've been holding out on me!'

'Me?' Red's cupped hands went to his chest in a gesture of innocence. 'Why, Malloy, I'm your friend!'

'Friend, hell!' Malloy shot back. 'You've been givin' me rotten stuff all along, and you just made a mistake and gave me some o'your good stuff. Now don't argue. This stuff you just gave me's got a *real* flavour. From now on, I want that, and none o' that other stuff.'

A hush fell over the place as the three plotters inhaled heavy sighs of relief. He wasn't suspicious after all—at least of what *they* had in mind. Tony quickly took advantage of the situation. He nodded, and Red poured Malloy another glass of wood alcohol.

At 1 o'clock next morning, Malloy, still at the bar drinking what people normally use in car radiators, suddenly crumpled in the middle, struck his chin on the edge of the bar, and crashed to the floor. The three plotters ran to the prostrate form, and examined him.

Pasqua, knowing not a little about the human body, put his hand over Malloy's heart. 'He's about gone,' he said with a sinister smile. 'It's barely beating.'

The trio laid Malloy out on a couch in the rear room, then sat around to wait for death.

An hour passed, and Malloy's heartbeat grew stronger! At 3 a.m., the 'murder victim' stirred perceptibly. At 6 a.m. he was fully awake, bounding from the couch like a child eager for play.

'More of that good alky, lad!' he yelled, running to the bar.

Tony and the undertaker ducked out of view. Red alone remained to make explanations. When Malloy noticed that it was daylight, he drunkenly asked what had happened, and Red replied that Malloy had had one too many and had fallen asleep.

Night after night, Malloy dropped into the speakeasy and, under the watchful eyes of the murder trust, was administered enough wood alcohol to kill, it seemed to them, a dozen strong, healthy men—let alone a man like Malloy. But night after night, much to the trio's chagrin, Malloy would merely fold up, take a nose-dive and a nap, then wake up as strong as ever with the break of day.

It need hardly be said that the murder trust was by now searching for a more potent means of dispatch.

Nor were they long in finding it. Red, had once hoped to become a chemist, so he knew all about ptomaine poisoning. He knew, for instance, that canned fish, if left in the tin, would produce that particularly type of illness, as he told Tony Marino.

'So why don't we open a can of them sardines on the shelf—we never sell 'em anyway—let 'em stand around for a while, then make this guy a sandwich? That ought to get him.'

A gleam came into Tony's eyes, and he uttered his favourite expression: 'An idea. An idea.'

Tony was extravagant in some respects. He opened six cans of sardines instead of one. And disdaining to let them stand a day for fear that they would not become putrid enough, he ordered that they be laid aside for a week. He also decided that a different brand of anti-freeze be fed to Michael Mallory. In that way, it might not even be necessary to use the sardines.

A week passed, during which time, Malloy continued to ingest the profferred anti-freeze. But Marino was finally ready to prepare the sandwiches. He even gave them his personal attention.

Tony sliced the bread (rye, which Malloy preferred), buttered it, and spread on the poisoned fish. He looked at his handiwork, then thought of how immune Malloy had been to the wood alcohol, and decided upon a certain improvement.

He stuck one of the sardine tins in his pocket and vacated his speakeasy for 15 minutes. On his return, he took from his pocket a small brown packet and carefully unwrapped it. A glistening substance within, resembling silver, was carefully blended with the sardines in the sandwich. It was the finely-cut remains of one of the sardine cans. If that wouldn't fix Malloy nothing would!

That night, Michael Malloy, in addition to his drinks, was offered a free snack. The drunkard, accepting with gratitude, reached for the sandwich that Red held out on a cracked plate.

Malloy munched into it. Between bites, he reached for his anti-freeze 'straight,' commenting freely on the excellence of the food and the liquor.

Malloy finished the sandwich. There were no immediate ill-effects. But when he ambled out into the night, the conspirators were convinced that they would never see him alive again. That ground tin would get him by morning at the latest.

But Malloy appeared the next night, asking for the usual alky, and more sandwiches. There being nothing but some innocuous 'baloney' on hand, he was given a sandwich of that. Red, man of science, walked into the rear room and attempted to cheer Tony, who made no effort to conceal his disappointment over the impotence of his last bit of macabre handiwork.

'If you've been drinkin',' Red suggested, 'and eat enough raw oysters, they turn to stone in your stomach and kill you.'

'This guy's awful tough,' said Tony. 'And he's beginnin' to get on my nerves. Now, if them oysters would kill him just from eatin' them, why wouldn't it be better to put them in some alky and soak them first!'

Next night, Malloy was fed a dozen raw oysters, pickled overnight in anti-freeze mixture. Malloy drowned them with his usual gusto, taking several gulps of the wood alcohol before and afterwards.

Once more Malloy proved the exception, rather than the rule, to an assault on the human constitution. If other people would have doubted up and died from consuming the ghastly mixture, Malloy was blissfully unaware of it. He sat around all that evening, downing more alcohol.

'This guy could eat arsenic,' remarked Tony to Pasqua and Red the next day. 'We gotta find another way.'

A few nights later, 'another way' was decided upon just before Malloy wandered in at his usual hour—9 p.m. Red's instructions that night were to get him thoroughly stiff. As usual, it took several hours to accomplish that.

Finally convinced that Malloy was completely 'out,' Tony and Pasqua carried him out and put him in a cab driven by one Hershey Green, another thoroughly disreputable character.

The unconscious Malloy was driven to the sprawling expanse of Claremont Park. It was one of the coldest nights of the winter and, as on the night that Malloy was first singled out as the victim of the murder plot, a violent sleet storm was pelting the city.

The undertaker, itching for a job, and Tony, his palm primed for the insurance money, jumped out of the cab, then looked up and down the street. There was not a soul in sight.

The two dragged Malloy's unconscious form from the cab, Tony grasping his arms, Pasqua his legs, slithered across the sleet-covered pavement with the victim, then disappeared into the forest of barren trees.

A hundred feet in from the street, they dropped the body, then stripped Malloy to the waist. Then Tony went back to the cab and returned with a demijohn filled with ice water, which he poured over Malloy's chest to ensure that he would either die of exposure or contact pneumonia.

Next morning, Pasqua entered the speakeasy early. His throat was swathed in red flannel. He couldn't speak above a croak. He had contracted a severe throat cold during the sinister doings of the night before. Tony, too, wasn't feeling any too well. He was sneezing and coughing, and his eyes were red. 'What a way to make money,' he observed, 'riskin' your health.'

'Well,' answered Pasqua, 'we'll get over this—but HE won't.'

A little later, while Tony and the undertaker were commiserating with each other, the buzzer sounded. It was Malloy!

'Mornin', lad,' the derelict chirped to Red, rubbing his hands together. 'Got a bit of a chill last night. How about a quick shot of that alky of yours?'

To say that Tony and Pasqua looked on in amazement when they saw the hale and hearty Malloy is something of an understatement. The man seemed nothing short of indestructible.

The murder plot, unsuccessful as it was, was now running into time, loss of sleep, risk of health, and money. Marino was getting desperate, so he called in a specialist in homicide—an oversized lug who referred to himself, in all seriousness, as Tough Tony. His last name was Bastone.

Marino outlined his problem to Tough Tony, then asked the other's advice.

'All you gotta do,' said Tough Tony, with professional pride, 'is to get a car to run him over. That's an accident, and you get double for that.'

An accident! Double indemnity!

'An idea,' said Marino. 'An idea.'

They got Malloy thoroughly intoxicated again the following night, and in the early hours of the morning took him out to a deserted thoroughfare known as Gun Hill Road. There was no moon that night.

The unconscious Malloy was lifted from the cab by Marino and Tough Tony, with Pasqua and driver Hershey Green remaining in the car.

There was a meshing of gears, the crescendo of a speeded motor, and the cab was off in the darkness. It went up the road a quarter of a mile, then turned around and began to gather speed.

Presently a horn tooted twice – the signal to Marino and Tough Tony that the cab was coming back again. The two, bracing the inebriated Malloy, stepped out into the street as a pair of headlights came closer.

As the car approached at 40 miles an hour, Hershey Green chanced to notice a woman peering out of a bedroom window.

And so, as the others shoved Malloy into the centre of the road, Green swerved his cab sharply to the left to avoid running over the man in the presence of a witness.

The murder trust decided upon a change of scene. Thus, on

Baychester Avenue, some distance away, the stage for the kill was set again.

This time, when Green tooted his horn twice, no one save the killers heard it. Tough Tony propped up the limp form of Malloy and shoved it forward when the cab came scuttling forward at high speed.

Marino stood back in the shadows and grinned evilly as he saw Tough Tony step back just in time to avoid the streaking cab. But Malloy didn't escape. The car struck him with terrific impact, and its wheels went over his booze-sodden body.

Their work done for the night, the members of the murder trust went home to bed, leaving Malloy lying in the road. Next morning, they gathered early in Tony's speakeasy as Red bought the latest papers.

The plotters scanned the columns of all the newspapers, looking for a story about an unidentified man being found dead on Baychester Avenue, victim of a hit-and-run driver. They scanned in vain.

'What could have happened?' Marino inquired of the assembled group. Then, addressing Green, the taxi driver: 'You sure he wasn't still lyin' there when you looked this afternoon?' Green shook his head.

Pasqua was the next to speak. 'Sometimes the papers don't have space for all the news. Besides, this guy ain't what you'd call prominent. Nobody would be interested in him except us.'

It was decided that Malloy had been picked up and removed to a morgue, so Red was instructed to make the rounds of the various city morgues. He was told to be sure and look at every body brought in since Malloy's unfortunate 'accident.'

Red had news for the plotters when he walked into Tony's speakeasy late the following afternoon. He had been to every morgue in Great New York, looked at every stiff, and none of them was Malloy.

An expression of amazement crossed Marino's dark countenance 'You don't suppose,' he demanded, 'he's still alive, do you?'

Tough Tony opined that such was a possibility, and an air of gloom settled over the little room.

Marino then told Red: 'Go up the street to the drug store and start callin' the hospitals. Somethin' tells me he ain't dead.'

Red spent a long time in that telephone booth. When he came out, perspiring, he was the picture of dejection. At each hospital, it had been the same story—'No one by that name or description has been brought in. Have you tried the other institutions?'

Nothing short of desperate in his desire to collect the insurance money—almost two months had passed now since the gang first went to work on Malloy—Tony decided on a bold stroke. He would find a substitute for the man who couldn't be killed!

The plotters began a tour of the Harlem speakeasies, looking for a new victim. It was in a dive in the Scratch Park district of Harlem where Bastone saw, leaning against the bar in a fairly drunken condition, a man of the same general appearance as Malloy.

Tough Tony struck up a conversation with the stranger, whose name was Joe Murphy. He was homeless and jobless, which made him eligible. Tough Tony told him that a friend of his who ran a speakeasy needed a handyman. The pay would be a dollar a day, and all he could drink. Would Mr Murphy consider such an opportunity? Yes, Mr Murphy would.

Tough Tony scribbled down the address of Marino's dive, and Murphy showed up next day for work.

That night, the killers plied the prospective victim with smoke, and he soon succumbed. Tony planted a card bearing the name 'Michael Malloy' in the man's pocket, then hastily went about the grim business of murder.

On a desolate thoroughfare in the upper Bronx, the uncounscious Murphy was thrown in front of Hershey Green's cab and knocked down like a matchstick in a hurricane. They lingered this time, prepared to run Murphy over a second time if he was not already dead. But Pasqua, the undertaker, announced that Green had done his work well.

'You'll collect the insurance now,' he assured Marino.

Next day, however, it was apparent that something had gone awry again. Murphy's body had been removed, yet it had not been received at any of the morgues. Then came the bad news. A man registered as Michael Malloy had been picked up the night previously, and taken to Fordham Hospital. When Marino called at the institution, he learned that Murphy was not dead at all, but was suffering from a compound fracture of the skull, a broken ar, a fractured leg, several broken ribs, a severe injury to his right eye, exposure, and internal injuries.

That night, as the murder trust bemoaned their plight, the buzzer sounded. A familiar figure entered.

'Evenin', lad! I'm dyin' for a drink. Make it snappy!'

It was, of course, Michael Malloy.

Malloy had met with a slight accident, he announced, and had been taken to a hospital (one that Red had evidently neglected to call), suffering from minor bruises.

'There was really nothin' wrong with me,' he told Red, banging his glass on the bar for an encore. 'Just scratched up a bit. But they kept me there.' Malloy gulped down another glass of anti-freeze mixture. 'It's nice to be back, lad. Couldn't get any o' this in the hospital.'

Would the gang *ever* succeed in murdering Malloy? Wood alcohol, poisoned sardines, a ground-up sardine tin, oysters and anti-freeze mixture, a night spent half naked in a sleet storm, being run over—he had withstood every murderous onslaught. Not only that; he actually seemed to be thriving on the treatment he was getting!

Malloy's fate hung in the balance for the next few days. His vitality had thoroughly disgusted the plotters, but they were reluctant to make any further attempts on his life, believing that the second 'Malloy' would die of his injuries. When, however, it was learned at the hospital that Murphy was expected to recover (which he eventually did), the gang decided on just one more try at abruptly abbreviating Michael Malloy's journey through life.

Red rented a room in a boarding-house on Fulton Avenue, in the Bronx. On the afternoon of Washington's Birthday, he and a friend of the ring—Daniel Kriesberg, a financially-embarrassed fruit dealer— inveigled Malloy into visiting the room on the pretext of sampling a new brand of alcohol.

Malloy sampled to his heart's content, and presently fell into his not-unfamiliar state of unconsciousness. Kreisberg and Red lost no time. They brought out a length of brown rubber tubing, fastened it to a gas jet, turned on the gas, then put the other end of the tubing in Malloy's mouth. The unconscious derelict, filled with alcohol, was breathing heavily, which was ideal for the macabre business at hand.

They left the tube in Malloy's mouth for more than an hour. Then they removed it, shut off the gas, and Red stuck the tube in his pocket.

Michael Malloy, at long last, was dead!

Kreisberg left, and Hershey Green, the taxi driver, joined Red in the murder room. It was late in the afternoon, and Marino, the mastermind, had instructed that the two men remain with the body so that it wouldn't be discovered until arrangements could be made for its disposal.

Darkness fell with still no word from Tony. Green and Red, not daring to disobey, remained in the room with the corpse. All night long, as a feeble light cast a dull yellow glow on the body of Malloy, the two men sitting within a few feet of the corpse played cards.

In the morning, a doctor—we'll call him Arnold Blodgett, although that isn't his real name—an old friend of the undertaker arrived. He looked at the body, then issued a death certificate ascribing the demise to pneumonia.

The body was removed to Pasqua's undertaking establishment. Pasqua, out for all he could get, didn't even bother to embalm it. He placed it, clothed just as it was when death came in a crude pine box, not even stopping to remove a plug of chewing tobacco from the hip pocket.

Michael Malloy was interred in Ferncliffe Cemetery, and Tony Marino collected more than 1,200 dollars in insurance money. Tony kept most of it for himself, dividing the balance among Kreisberg, Pasqua, Red and Tough Tony Bastone.

Everything went along very smoothly for more than two months—with the exception of the murder of Tough Tony in Marino's speakeasy by a young man who suddenly sickened of Tony's constant exhibitions of toughness. This affair, however, had nothing to do with the murder of Michael Malloy. Until now—the early part of May—there had been no hint of suspicion in connection with the derelict's death.

Then one of the District Attorney's most able assistants—Edward Breslin—heard a rumour that an insurance murder had been committed in the Bronx some time previously. Breslin's information was of the most fragile sort, however. He had no names, no addresses, no date. All he learned was that the undertaker in the case had been an Italian.

Breslin got in touch with Bronx Detective Edward Byrness and told him the story.

Breslin and Byrnes first examined every death certificate issue in New York City for a period of six months, several thousand in all. In each instance, they immediately eliminated the certificate if the undertaker's name was not Italian. All certificates bearing such names were retained for future investigation.

It was a painstaking job, but it was about to bring results when detectives began to probe into what might lie behind the death certificate they found bearing the name of Michael Malloy, with Frank Pasqua as undertaker and Dr Arnold Blodgett as the attending physician.

When it was learned that Pasqua had done practically no business to speak of for some time, and that his reputation was none too savoury, Detective Byrnes' next move was to call at the house on Fulton Avenue where Malloy died. The death certificate had stated that it was a private residence, and Byrnes immediately noticed that it was a rooming-house. This at once increased suspicion, for it is a strict rule that everything a physician writes on a death certificate must be absolutely accurate.

Byrnes next communicated with various insurance companies, and learned that Tony Marino, the speakeasy proprietor, had been the beneficiary of an insurance policy issued on Malloy. And Byrnes immediately recalled the murder of Tough Tony Bastone in Marino's place.

Marino and his pals were shadowed night and day from that moment on. When it was noted that he and Pasqua were obviously more than casual friends, the investigation became more intense. Byrnes called at the rooming-house where Malloy died, interviewed the landlady, and asked who had rented the room. The woman, an honest soul with nothing to hide, said that Mr Malloy's brother had. This was a new lead, for the insurance policy had stated that Malloy was homeless.

'Do you remember what Malloy's brother looked like?' asked Byrnes.

'I remember him very well,' the landlady answered, 'because he had such bright red hair. He was not a nice-looking man. In fact, I was a little afraid of him.'

'How old would you say he was?'

'Oh, about 30.'

The woman had described Red the bartender.

The whole gang was carefully watched now, and an order was issued to exhume Michael Malloy's body. As already stated, Pasqua hadn't bothered to embalm it—and that's where he made a fatal mistake. Embalming fluid would have removed the high pink colouring that is the result of death by gas. But now, after all these months, the corpse (remarkably preserved, by the way, owing to Malloy's constant indulgence in alcohol) was as pink as it had been the morning after death. There could be no question as to the cause of death.

It was at this stage of the investigation that a clerk in the District Attorney's office recalled a singular fact. This man, as a reporter on the *New York World*, had, three years previously, worked on the story of the death of Maybelle Carlson, the blonde streetwalker found in her room, nude and the windows open, in mid-winter. And the ex-reporter now recalled that none other than Tony Marino had been the beneficiary named in Miss Carlson's insurance policy.

The gang was rounded up. On October 21st, 1933, the four arch-plotters—Tony Marino, Red Murphy, Pasqua, the murdering undertaker, and Kreisberg, who with Red, was one of the actual slayers—were sentenced to death in the electric chair at Sing Sing. The following year, on June 8th, 1934, Kreisberg, Marino and Pasqua were executed. Red Murphy won a stay of execution, but less than a month later, on July 6th, he followed the others to the chair.

Meanwhile, Hershey Green, the taxi driver, had pleaded guilty to the charge of assault and was sentenced to serve five to 10 years in prison. Dr Blodgett, the last figure in the case, was acquitted of being an accessory, but was found guilty of failing to report a suspicious death, for which he served a brief prison term.

JOHN LAWRENCE
Murder for Murder's Sake

'I want to be known as the greatest criminal that ever lived,' declared Jane Toppan. 'That is my ambition.'

She succeeded in her ambition. The story of her crimes is almost incredible.

In the middle 'sixties a Mrs Anne Toppan, of Lowell, in the United States, adopted a little girl, Nora Kelly, the daughter of Peter Kelly, a bit of a wastrel. Later, Nora Kelly, whose name had been changed to Jane Toppan, was brought up by a daughter of Mrs Anne Toppan, a Mrs Brigham. Years later Mrs Brigham died suddenly, as did her sister.

Jane Toppan was a remarkably pretty child with big black eyes, fair skin and dark hair. She was famous for her high spirits and constant laughter. She had the reputation, indeed, of being the most merry-hearted child in all Lowell. Her foster parents were well-to-do, and their adopted child was sent to the Lowell High School to be educated. She was not trained for any particular profession, for apart from her parents being rich enough to leave her well provided for, there was every prospect that a girl of her attractiveness and high spirits would get married.

In her early 'twenties Jane Toppan became engaged, but her engagement did not last very long. Her lover not only broke it off suddenly, but within a short time had married another girl. From that day Jane Toppan changed. Unhappy, doubly unhappy from having nothing to do, she expressed a wish to become a hospital nurse, and entered the Cambridge Hospital at the age of twenty-five. In hospital she proved at first to be one of the best nurses that had been trained there for a long time, quick, intelligent, skilful, and eager to learn all she could, especially about the effects of certain medicines and drugs. But it was in the

Cambridge Hospital that the first signs of her loss of balance began to show itself.

Under her charge was a young man who was puzzling the doctor. When the patient should have been on the high road to recovery, and indeed was, his temperature, as recorded on Nurse Toppan's chart, remained persistently above normal. The doctor, completely puzzled, at last took his patient's temperature himself and to his astonishment he found it to be perfectly normal. Nurse Toppan was called to account, and confessed that she had fallen in love with her patient and had falsified the temperature sheet so that he should be kept in hospital and under her care.

She was dismissed from the hospital and went to the Massachusetts General Hospital in Boston, where she completed her course without raising any suspicion that she was in any way abnormal. When she left the hospital she was soon in demand, and began to take charge of cases in the best families in Cambridge. At that time she made her home in a cottage, about a quarter of a mile from Harvard. The cottage belonged to the Dunham family, and in that cottage death began to be Nurse Toppan's companion.

Nurse Toppan was a great favourite of Israel Dunham and his wife, for although in some respects she had become harder, she had not lost that smile which had characterised her since she was a child. She was always smiling, and was a great favourite with children. No one, indeed, suspected this smiling nurse of a grudge against mankind, a grudge so bitter, so secret, that it was not suspected until she had murdered at least thirty people, and probably many more.

On May 26th, 1895, Israel Dunham died suddenly at his home in Cambridge. He had been suffering from hernia, and was nursed by Jane Toppan. The doctor had no hesitation in giving a death certificate. He had no reason to suspect that the smiling nurse had given her patient an overdose of morphine, for the sole reason that she thought he was too old to live. In September, 1897, Mrs Dunham was taken ill and her death on the 19th of that month was put down to heart failure. So it was, but not the kind of heart failure the doctor who signed the death certificate had in mind.

For a time Jane Toppan acted as nurse at the hospital of the theological seminary at Cambridge. The matron, Mrs Myra Connor, died from a complication of ailments. She was assiduously nursed by Nurse Toppan who, on her death, took her place as matron. But she did not hold the position for long. Life was too dull in the hospital of a theological seminary to suit Jane Toppan.

It will be recalled that when her foster mother, Mrs Anne Toppan died, Jane had been brought up by the former's married daughter, Mrs Brigham, and her husband, whom she had learnt to call father and mother. Jane had not seen the Brighams for some years, although she had been very fond of her foster father. But for Mrs Brigham she had conceived a violent dislike, for she believed that Mrs Brigham had robbed her of some money which she thought she ought to have had under the will of Mrs Anne Toppan. Nurse Toppan had very successfully concealed her hatred, but it smouldered in her brain for years, and when, in 1899, Mr and Mrs Brigham came to visit her in a cottage she had at Cataumet, on Buzzard's Bay, the murdering nurse saw her opportunity and seized avidly upon it.

On August 29th, 1899, Mrs Brigham died at the age of sixty-one after a two days' illness, and the doctor gave a certificate for 'heart failure due to cerebral apoplexy.' A good many persons Jane Toppan nursed died from 'heart failure.'

Jane accompanied the body back to her old home at Lowell. The day of the funeral she went smiling about the old house, and when Mr Brigham, who had been very fond of his wife, remonstrated, she replied that she was only trying to keep cheerful because she loved him and did not want to see him too downhearted. Mr Brigham did not realize that his foster daughter really did love him and had already begun to hate the housekeeper, a Miss Calkins. She strongly suspected that Mr Brigham meant to marry his housekeeper later on, and Nurse Toppan took immediate steps to prevent such an occurrence. In January Miss Calkins was taken ill, and on the fifteenth of the month, 1900, she died.

After the death of his housekeeper Mr Brigham asked his married sister, Mrs Bannister, to come and live with him. This was exactly what Nurse Toppan did not want. She wanted Mr Brigham to herself. Mrs Bannister stood in her way, and Jane had her own methods of removing obstacles. Mrs Bannister had never been a very strong woman, but when she came to stay with her brother her ailments increased. She went from bad to worse, and died on August 27th, 1900. Afterwards it was shown that she had died from morphine poisoning.

Mr Brigham asked no one else to come and stay with him, though he suspected nothing. But he sent Jane Toppan back to her cottage at Cataumet. She did not stay there long. Early in 1901 some old friends of hers, a Mr and Mrs Davis, invited her to stay with them at their cottage on Buzzard's Bay. The cottage was only one in name. Actually it had once been a hotel of twenty rooms, and in this house there were only staying Mr and Mrs Davis, Jane Toppan, and a servant.

As the warm weather of June came Mrs Davis began to complain of feeling ill. She had been troubled with kidney disease for some years and her illness was put down to this cause. She was advised to have a change of air, and Jane Toppan suggested that she might like to come and stay with her in Cambridge. They arrived there on June 27th, but the change of air seemed to have a very bad effect on the old lady. She rapidly became worse, and died on July 4th, 1901. The doctor gave the cause of death as diabetes.

It was supposed that Mrs Davis had a large sum of money in a purse, but it was not found after her death, nor was it known for some time afterwards that Nurse Toppan had borrowed considerable sums of money from the old lady and had not repaid them.

The extraordinary fact is that still no one suspected the smiling nurse. She was, indeed, very popular with everyone, so much so that when Mrs Davis died Mr Davis invited her to come and stay with him and his married daughters, a Mrs Harry Gordon and a Mrs Minnie Gibbs. By this invitation he was to encompass his own death as well as those of his daughters. Both Mr Davis and Mrs Gordon had lent the nurse money, for which the latter had given I.O.U's. Neither of them, however, were pressing her for the return of their loans, for both were comparatively well-to-do. But the smiling nurse conceived the idea that if they died she would never have to repay the money she owed. There was another reason why Mrs Gordon was marked out for death. Nurse Toppan had made several unsuccessful attempts to get married and now she was to make another. She conceived the idea that if Mrs Gordon were dead that the latter's husband, Mr Harry Gordon, would marry her. Mrs Gordon was not feeling very well one night, but she felt decidedly worse after some medicine which Nurse Toppan persuaded her to take. A few nights afterwards she became seriously ill.

'I got up and worked over her to make others think I was anxious to have Mrs Gordon get well,' said Nurse Toppan in her confession, surely the most amazing confession ever made by a murderess. 'But she kept on sinking until she died on the morning of July 29th. I went to the funeral and felt as jolly as could be.'

'I had already begun to think how to get rid of Mr Davis. Somehow I didn't like him. I was afraid of him, though I didn't know why. He had been a friend of mine for years. I was afraid he would find out I had killed his wife and daughter. At first, after his wife's death, I thought he would marry me, but I found out he wouldn't, but might leave me some property in his will.'

Nurse Toppan wasn't particular whom she married, so long as it was someone with money. She had got her eye on Harry Gordon as a second string as soon as she began to feel that Mr Davis was not susceptible to her charms. But he might leave her some property, and that would come in useful when she did get married.

'Mr Davis went to Boston one hot day,' to quote from her confession, 'and when he came back he was pretty tired and almost prostrated. I saw my chance then, for I could say, if anyone suggested that he was poisoned, that he got the drug in Boston and committed suicide out of grief for his wife. The next day he was dead and they buried him beside his wife and daughter at the Cataumet Cemetery.'

The doctor put down the death of Mr Davis to heat apoplexy.

There is one remarkable sentence in Nurse Toppan's confession which I cannot forbear from quoting here.

'I made it lively for the undertakers and grave-diggers that time,' she said. 'Three graves in a little over three weeks in one lot in the cemetery.'

In each case she had used her favourite poison, morphine, a poison which is not easy to detect and has the effect of weakening the heart's action. Wherever she could, Nurse Toppan chose for the time to administer the poison just when her victims were not feeling too well from perfectly natural causes. Mr Davis had come back from Boston really overcome by the heat, and everyone remarked how ill he looked. No surprise was expressed, therefore, when he died suddenly.

'Then I turned my attention to the last surviving member of the Davis family, Mrs Irving Minnie Gibbs.'

Minnie Gibbs was looked upon as being Nurse Toppan's best friend. The two had known one another for many years and there had never been any quarrel between them. But there are many cases where people have turned upon their best friends, and Nurse Toppan was no exception. From Minnie, as from the rest of the family, Jane Toppan had borrowed money. And again, as with the murder of Mrs Gordon, there was a man in the offing. If Gordon did not marry her there was always Mr Gibbs—if he were a widower.

'This is just how I poisoned Minnie Gibbs. We all went driving to

Woods Hall one day, and when we came back Minnie was not feeling well. I had given her a morphia tablet dissolved in hot whisky before we started 'to brace her up for the drive' I said to her.

' "You had better take some of Dr Latter's medicine,' I said on our return, but she said she did not want any medicine. I insisted that she should have it, and I gave her some with morphia tablets dissolved in it.'

In the night Nurse Toppan got up and found that Mrs Gibbs was still living, and to make sure she should not see another dawn she gave her an injection of morphia.

Mrs Gibbs died on August 13, 1901. It was the last of the terrible series of murders by this modern Lucrezia Borgia. For years she had violated the almost sacred relationship of nurse and patient. The motives of former women poisoners—and woman have been the greatest poisoners in history—have not as a rule been complex. Lucrezia Borgia murdered from ambition or revenge. Catherine de Medici adopted this method of ridding herself of human obstacles for similar reasons, and the Marquise de Brinvilliers poisoned her father, two brothers, her child and others in order to enrich himself.

But Jane Toppan eclipsed them all in the number and horror of her crimes, and seems largely to have murdered for the sheer pleasure of killing. At times it seemed as though she had killed because her victim was an obstacle in the way of her marriage, but though she put forward that as an excuse, she certainly was chameleonlike in her rapid changes of possible husbands. Mrs Davis died on July 4th, 1901. As Mr Davis had shown no inclination to marry his wife's murderess almost immediately after the funeral she lost patience and Mr Davis himself was dead before the month was out. So was Mrs Gordon, his daughter, and when Harry Gordon did not respond, Nurse Toppan's greatest friend died, and she turned her attention to her greatest friend's husband, Mr Gibbs.

Jane Toppan had been murdering a little too rapidly in that July and August. Four people in less than two months began to make those left alive talk. And once the tongue of rumour began wagging there was no stopping it. Rumour at last became so strong that the police were forced to take action. The body of Mrs Gibbs was exhumed and the internal organs were analysed by Professor Wood, of Harvard University, for poison. He discovered that the body of Mrs Gibbs contained no less than ten grains of morphine and a similar amount of atropine. The authorities lost no time in taking action, once the fact that one of Nurse

Toppan's patients had been poisoned was established. They had had before them a list of the last half a dozen patients of hers who had died suddenly, and they were determined to arrest her before any more of her patients passed away with appalling swiftness. Post mortem examinations were carried out on Mr and Mrs Davis, and in both cases, from the amount of poison found in their bodies, it was abundantly clear that both had died from exactly the same cause as Mrs Gibbs.

Nurse Toppan's arrest revealed a horrible, terrifying story, only the very barest outlines of which have been already given. She had a diseased mind, which was only satisfied by the killing of people whom she disliked or who she felt were better out of the way. After her arrest, and when the story of her crimes were gradually becoming known, it was soon obvious that she must have been made for years, though, with that remarkable cunning of mad people, she had successfully hidden it. Her last four murders were merely the culminating point of a brain already beginning to break down completely. She was examined by three of the leading alienists in America, all of whom pronounced her insane. In the face of their evidence the jury brought in a verdict of 'Guilty, but insane,' and she was sent to Taunton Asylum for the insane. And there she wrote out a confession which began by denying her insanity, but which, by the sheer horror of it, proves it. The confession is one which would not have been credited normally, but practically everything she said in it was confirmed from outside sources.

'The easiest way out of it,' she wrote, 'was to be judged insane, I thought, and sent to an asylum. Then I could get out again after a while, perhaps, when all this excitement about my case had died down and the doctors would say I was 'cured.'

'When the famous insanity experts of Boston, Dr Jelly, Dr Stedman and Dr Quinby, came to see if I was insane, I knew how to fool them. I have been a trained nurse for fifteen years and know doctors and just how to manage them. I know what the opening remark of an insane person is to the doctors who are examining them. It is, 'I am not insane.' It is a queer thing but people who are really insane will always deny it. So I said to the alienists, 'I am not insane.'

'I knew I could fool them all. Dr Jelly and the other doctors tried me hard with many questions. They tried to play on my woman's sympathy and asked me if I didn't think it was a terrible thing to take those mothers, Mrs Gibbs and Mrs Gordon, away from their young children. But I knew their game, and said that I had killed them but I didn't know why. I killed them for various reasons, but it always gave me the most exquisite pleasure to see them die. They said, 'You must have been insane to have done such a thing.' But I still insisted that I was not insane and did not want them to make me out insane. Then they went away and gave their verdict that I was insane, which was just what I wanted.'

When Jane Toppan's confession was published many actually believed the doctors had been fooled and clamoured for her execution! But to the expert the whole of the beginning of this confession was a proof of her madness. Like most mad people, particularly those who are mad upon only one point, Jane Toppan could write and argue seemingly quite rationally on most subjects.

In some ways, in fact, the murderess was above the average in intelligence and ability. She was an omnivorous reader and a writer as well. While she was sitting beside her patients, often waiting for them to die, she would write short stories. One habit which she had was to read items aloud from the newspapers to her patients, and if the news was of some romance or tragedy, she would expand upon it and remark that it made a wonderful plot for a story. She was continually saying that some day she would give up nursing and write a really great novel. Actually when she was in prison waiting for trial she devoted all her time to writing this novel and told everyone that when it was published it would make her so rich that she would be able to pay all her lawyers fees for getting her out of prison.

The callousness of Jane Toppan's confession has never been equalled. Speaking of Mrs Davis, she wrote that Mrs Davis had fainted after running to catch a train. 'I saw this would be a good time to put her out of the way, and it would look as if she died of heart failure. I took her to my cottage. I was quite alone with my patient. After I had given Mrs Davis some lunch and told her to drink a little Hunyadi water that I had drugged with morphia, we went for a walk. But on the way she fainted. I saw that my medicine was working. She really was suffering from diabetes. She lingered along for ten days and all I needed to do was to give her just enough poison to help the disease to do its work quickly.'

Jane Toppan owed her long freedom from suspicion because she chose the right time to put her patients out of the way. Mr Davis, for example, had been suffering from the heat and the dose of morphia Jane Toppan gave him was sufficient to make the doctors believe he had had a heatstroke.

'People say I have no heart, but I have. While I have been in prison a friend in Lowell sent me some forget-me-nots and I cried. They were the flowers that my first lover used to send me when I was a schoolgirl. And a forget-me-not was engraved on the ring he gave me. He broke off the engagement and it seemed that my whole light-hearted nature changed after that. I still laughed and was jolly, but I learned how to hate, too. Some people have said I was a morphia fiend. I never took a morphia tablet in my life. I know its terrible effects too well.'

Here she spoke the truth. Altogether she confessed to having murdered thirty-one people, some out of sheer wantonness because she wanted to experiment with morphia and atropia so that she would know exactly the right doses to give to those people who stood in her way. Actually Nurse Toppan probably murdered more than fifty persons altogether, for the records of her cases showed over that number who had died more suddenly than the doctors had expected. All had been suffering from some ailment or another, and the smiling nurse worked so hard for them that she was never for one moment suspected. It is difficult to see how she could have been so long as she chose her victims carefully. It was when she made the mistake of trying to poison a whole family that she came under suspicion.

But confinement in the Taunton Lunatic Asylum brought about a change in Jane Toppan. Little by little she lost that smiling jollity which had earned her the nickname of the 'Jolly Poisoner.' She began to brood and to think that all the food which she had was poisoned. Within two years of entering the asylum as a plump, happy looking woman, she had become a thin, haggard reflection of her former self, a woman haunted by the horrors of her past, crazed by the fear that she was being given morphia by the nurses who looked after her. Her torments became so great at last that she became violent and had to be confined in a padded cell, round which she paced shrieking, 'Help, help, they are poisoning me.'

So great was her fear that she was to suffer the same fate of her own many victims, that she refused at last to take food at all, and had to be forcibly fed.

Finally, before her death, she got the delusion that her victims had all come to life again and were in the padded cell with her, taunting her with their deaths, describing their own tortures and the tortures she would suffer in her turn.

To Jane Toppan, the greatest woman poisoner who ever lived, death must have been a merciful release.

HAROLD EATON
Poison in a Private School

Since the days of the Borgias, poison has always been a favourite weapon of the 'gentleman' murderer. The more subtle the drug, the more secret the administration of it, the greater the artistic triumph. Knowledge of the properties of the various poisons postulates a certain mental ability, and so in a general way it may be said that the great poisoners have belonged to the educated classes. Palmer was a man of some social position; Crippen, Pritchard, and Lamson, the subject of this sketch, all had medical qualifications and possessed a considerable degree of culture; while even Seddon achieves a certain gentility through the method he employed to gain his ends.

Dr George Henry Lamson seems to have been born with a genius for friendship, and to have acquired a reputation for humanity. In 1876 and 1877 he served as a volunteer army-surgeon in Servia and Rumania, and in recognition of his work numerous decorations of both countries were conferred, upon him. Not only in England, but in America and on the Continent, he possessed a wide circle of friends, whose efforts to save him after conviction testified to the sincerity of their affection. He was a French scholar, could speak other European tongues, and had read much in many languages; in effect a young man of experience and promise, a young man whose generous impulses sometimes led him into extravagances, but all the same, a young man, it was thought, who would sober down one day and make his mark in the world. That his name will live for some while yet in the memory of man, seems to be assured.

In 1876, when he was in his twenty-sixth year, this young man of promise married. His wife, a Miss John, was a ward in Chancery, and upon marriage became entitled to a small fortune which, since the Married Women's Property Act was not then law, passed under the control of her husband. Among the new relations that this alliance brought to Lamson must be noticed Herbert John and Percy John, his wife's brothers, and Mrs Chapman, her sister. In 1879 Herbert John died suddenly under circumstances which, though they aroused no suspicion at the time, seem to indicate that the crime for which he was executed was not Lamson's first murder. At all events, through the death of her brother, Mrs Lamson became entitled to some £700, and with this money her husband purchased a medical practice in Bournemouth.

As a doctor, Lamson was unsuccessful, and his circumstances went from bad to worse, until finally the home was sold up. In April, 1881, he went to America; but whatever venture he attempted out there met with no better fortune than had his practice at Bournemouth, and he actually arrived back in England with nothing save £5 borrowed from the surgeon on board. That he was in desperate need of money there can be no doubt. A few pounds might still be borrowed, were, in fact, borrowed from friends; but his friends, though willing to help, were not rich. A large sum, a thousand pounds or more, were needed to square Lamson's debts and to set him upon his feet again.

It is possible to trace the mental processes that induced this young man, with a reputation for humanity and a genius for friendship, to turn in his search for money, first to fraud and forgery and finally to the gravest crime known to the law. Some years earlier he had become addicted to the morphine habit, contracted while serving in the Balkans, and he himself attributed his downfall to this cause. Probably his failure as a doctor was due to the drug, which disinclines the mind for a punctual routine of work; probably also his ethical preception was blurred by the use of the needle. It is charitable to suppose that the latter proposition, at all events, is true, for it may serve to palliate in some small measure what was possibly the most cunning and diabolical crime of the nineteenth century.

Without any very extravagant tastes, Lamson was yet not accustomed to stinting himself, and his generosity urged him to treat his friends more lavishly than his means warranted. He had now to provide for a wife and child, but his addiction to morphine prevented him pursuing any ordered and regular business. That had been tried and had failed. Experience and skill in his profession he certainly had, but he was unable to subdue the lethargy from which all drug-takers suffer. What, then, was to be done? Debtors were pressing and friends were not so staunch and cordial as they had been; were, in fact, disclined to lend money without any security whatsoever.

Other means must be found. He had still a banking account—overdrawn, it must be admitted—but he could write cheques which by some remote chance might be honoured. Moreover, his medical qualifications inspired tradesmen with a certain amount of confidence and induced them to grant credit up to a point. Small sums could be obtained in this way—not quite honestly, perhaps, but one never knew whether a bank was bluffing or not when it declared that no further cheques would be met.

These minor successes were all very well, but they were only temporary measures. In the end he grew more reckless, and, as will be shown later, he drew and cashed a cheque for £12 10s. upon a bank at which he had never had an account, though it is probable that at that time he had resolved upon murder, and was trying to provide himself with the money necessary to leave England. If he was still debating the issue, the difficulty which had attended this fraud and the paltry proceeds of it determined him. He had committed an offence for which he might receive a severe sentence, and what had he gained by it? A dozen pounds. These petty dishonesties were not worth while, were unworthy of his talents. What was needed was a big coup.

This excursion into crime was dangerous and amateurish enough: fraud, it would seem, was not his métier. Yet money had to be obtained from somewhere. He hadn't had much luck in the course of his life; just one slice and one slice only—the legacy from Herbert John.

The day before his execution, Lamson, while confessing that he had been rightly convicted, vehemently denied that he had been in any way concerned in the death of Herbert John. If for the moment we accept this statement, the fatal illness of his brother-in-law must have appeared to Lamson as an extremely opportune accident—an accident which, unfortunately, could not be repeated. Was there no one else by whose death he might hope to profit?

The answer was not far to seek. Were the other brother-in-law, Percy Malcolm John, to die unmarried and before attaining the age of twenty-one, half the £3000 which he would inherit upon either of these contingencies would pass to Mrs Lamson.

At the time of his death in 1881, Percy John was eighteen and was living at Blenheim House School, Wimbledon. A cripple from birth, he suffered from curvature of the spine and his lower limbs were paralysed.

He had, therefore, to propel himself about in a wheel-chair and to rely upon his school-fellows to carry him up and downstairs. Apart from his disability he seems to have enjoyed good health and to have possessed a cheerful disposition, which secured him many friends. His holidays he frequently passed with Dr Lamson and his sister, to whom he was devotedly attached. That he would live long was improbable, for the curvature was growing worse, but it was equally improbable that he would die in time to save Lamson from bankruptcy, perhaps from prison.

One can imagine that the doctor watched impatiently the slow progress of the disease, until at last his desperate need of money tempted him to assist nature. The boy could only live a few more years at most, could find but little in life to enjoy. Would not death be a merciful release?

Whether so humane a sophistry entered his mind, or whether the use of morphia had indeed distorted his sense of proportion to the point of madness, is a problem in psychology that can find no answer. Having made up his mind, he certainly set about his task with the proverbial cunning of the maniac. With the resources of science at his command he was able to choose a rare and subtle poison which, had he used it more moderately, might have escaped detection and defied any chemical tests known to the analysts of those days.

The weapon which he selected was aconitine, which is the active principle of the plant called 'Monks-hood' or 'Wolf's-bane,' and among the whole range of poisons he could have found nothing more deadly nor more horrible. There is no other recorded case of a murderer employing this drug by itself, and it is as the pioneer of a novel poison that Lamson's name will be remembered.

After his return from America in the summer of 1881, Lamson went to the Isle of Wight, and it was there that he made his first attempt upon the life of Percy John. The boy had come to spend his holidays with his sister at Shanklin, and there is little doubt that during his visit his brother-in-law administered a dose of aconitine to him under the guise of a quinine pill. Whether this was by way of experiment or whether Lamson thought that nature required only a little assistance, is uncertain. At all events, the boy completely recovered, and Lamson, grateful, perhaps, that he had failed, and hoping for some other means of rescue, made no further attempt until the following December. A second trip to America intervened, but it was as unsuccessful as the previous one, and he returned absolutely penniless, even being forced to pawn his watch and chain and a case of surgical instruments for £5.

If after his initial failure he had abandoned his design against his brother-in-law, the urgency of procuring money without delay reinstated the thought in his mind. Money he must have at all costs and, save for fraud and burglary, arts in which he had never graduated, there was no other way. In November, 1881, he was staying at Nelson's Hotel, Great Portland Street, and on the 20th he tried to purchase aconitine from Messrs. Bell & Co., in Oxford Street, but they refused to supply him on the ground that he was unknown to them. Nevertheless, on the 24th he managed to buy two grains of the poison from Messrs. Allen & Hanbury, and the ease with which he procured it was made the subject of a comment by the judge and of a recommendation by the jury. All he did—all, in fact, he was required to do by the Poisons Act—was to give his name and address, and without verifying his assertion that he was a doctor, the assistant handed over to him poison sufficient to kill thirty people. Recent cases emphasise the fact that poison—especially arsenic—is a component part of many commodities, from which it can easily be separated, and it seems desirable that some more drastic restrictions should be introduced.

Having made his preparations, Lamson tried to obtain funds to keep him going until he could put his plan into execution. On November 26th he went to the American Exchange office and asked them to cash a cheque on the Wilts. and Dorset Bank for £15. This the exchange refused to do. Three days later, Lamson, though lacking the money for the fare, managed to get to Ventnor by assuring the railway authorities that his friends there would reimburse them. His idea in going to the Isle of Wight was, no doubt, to try to raise money in a place where he and his family were known, but where the news of his acute poverty had not so far penetrated. In this he was partially successful, and induced Mr Price Owen to advance him £20 upon a cheque drawn on the Wilts. and Dorset Bank.

Once the money was in his possession and his fare to London assured, Lamson realised that what he had done amounted probably to the offence of obtaining money by false pretences. He knew well enough that the cheque was worthless and that Mr Owen would discover that fact in a day or two. Time must be gained somehow. Accordingly he wired to his victim:

> JUST DISCOVERED THAT CHEQUE YOU ASKED YESTER-
> DAY MADE ON WRONG BANK. PLEASE DON'T SEND IT ON.
> LETTER FOLLOWS.

The letter, written from his hotel in London, explained the mistake plausibly and circumstantially. He had formerly had an account at the Wilts. and Dorset Bank, but had transferred his business elsewhere. Still retaining a few blank cheques upon the former bank, he had stupidly mixed up his old cheque book with his new one. He had wired for the right cheque book and would put the matter straight as soon as it arrived.

Lamson must long before have decided that the murder of Percy John was the only solution of his difficulties, but the safest and swiftest method of administrating the poison remained to be considered. In a few weeks the boy would be coming to spend his Christmas holidays with him. Should he do it then? He could announce that his brother-in-law, never strong, was ill; he would, of course, be the boy's medical attendant, could, if necessary, counterfeit symptoms and even sign the certificate of death. Small risk of detection here! And yet, the delay—three weeks! How was he to support himself for those three weeks; how to adjust those little money matters which smelt so strongly of fraud? In any event, it would be a month or two before he would actually receive his wife's share of the boy's estate, but it would be easy to borrow upon his expectations as soon as his brother-in-law was dead. There must be no more hesitation, no more half-hearted, bungling measures such as that first attempt of his at Shanklin in the summer. The deed should be done surely and immediately.

Yet this man who had chosen the most subtle of poisons and who had so long pondered over his plans, committed the actual crime so clumsily that he at once fastened suspicion on himself. Perhaps his eagerness betrayed him, perhaps his addiction to morphine prevented him from paying proper attention to detail. He had been a failure in fraud and now, with every chance of an artistic triumph, he was to become a slipshod murderer.

Having decided to act without delay, he had next to consider what was the best method of administering the poison—a problem that presented few difficulties to one skilled in medicine and possessing the complete confidence of his victim. One other matter still remained to be settled and that was his conduct after the commission of the crime. Should he return to London and await quietly the painful news of his brother-in-law's sudden death? His nerves were strong, but were they strong enough for that? Was he a good enough actor to sympathise convincingly with his wife's grief and to conceal all signs of satisfaction and eagerness? It would perhaps be safer to leave England for a short time, in case anything untoward occurred, and to claim the £1500 upon his return.

On December 1st he visited a medical student called John Tulloch, a great friend of his, and announced that he would shortly be going to Paris. That he published this news to anyone else, except Mr Bedbrook, the schoolmaster, seems uncertain, but no doubt he wished to convey a general impression that he had long ago decided to visit Paris, and he cunningly made this trip of his an excuse for going to see Percy John. So affectionate a brother-in-law would naturally wish to say good-bye to the boy—even though he might only be absent a few weeks.

> 'MY DEAR PERCY,' he wrote, 'I had intended running down to Wimbledon to see you today, but I have been delayed by various matters until it is now nearly six o'clock, and by the time I should reach Blenheim House you would probably be preparing for bed. I leave for Paris and Florence to-morrow and wish to see you before going, so I purpose to run down to your place as early as I can for a few minutes, even if I can accomplish no more. Believe me, my dear boy, your loving brother,
> 'GEORGE LAMSON.'

This was written on December 1st, and had he succeeded in putting his schemes into execution the next evening, he would doubtless have left for Paris as stated in the letter. His subsequent excuse that Mr Bedbrook had told him that there was a bad boat running that night and that he had therefore modified his original plans, was utterly false and became not the weakest link in the chain of suspicion that ultimately led to his arrest.

On December 2nd he went down to Wimbledon with Tulloch, and, leaving his friend at a public house, went off, ostensibly to call at the school. That he never visited Blenheim House on that evening is one of the curious features of the case, and the reason for this manœuvre seems obscure. It may be that his heart failed him, or may be that he had forgotten some essential part of his rôle of poisoner. At all events, he rejoined Tulloch after an absence of twenty minutes and told him that he had seen his brother-in-law, and that the poor boy was manifestly weaker. His mournful prophecy that Percy John would not last much longer cannot, perhaps, be cited as an authentic example of clairvoyance.

Probably lack of funds made him withhold his hand upon that day. He had committed himself to a trip abroad, but it is doubtful whether he had sufficient money for the fare. If possible, he must raise the wind just once more in order to induce that long-desired windfall.

He returned to town with Tulloch, and the pair went to the Comedy Theatre in Panton Street. Subsequently Lamson drew a cheque in favour of his friend, whom he asked to cash it for him. As this cheque was upon a bank at which the doctor had not then and never had had an account, this action constituted a grave criminal offence. No doubt he anticipated that the cheque would be returned marked 'No account,' and that by then he would have borrowed from some other source sufficient to satisfy Tulloch. The idea of an immediate loan as soon as Percy John was dead must have been one of the chief factors in his schemes, for Tulloch, in spite of their friendship, and in spite of the fact that he and Lamson were rarely out of one another's debt, does not appear to have been the sort of man who would have tried to hush up this transaction.

Ultimately, after a rebuff at the Adelphi Hotel, they succeeded in cashing the cheque at the Eyre Arms, St John's Wood, and Lamson, with the means of escape in his pocket, had now no reason to hesitate or to delay.

The following evening, a few minutes before seven o'clock, he called at Blenheim House and asked to see Percy John. The latter was carried upstairs to the dining-room, where he found Lamson and Mr Bedbrook, the headmaster, and the three of them sat there chatting for some minutes. That the mental strain of the last few months had told upon the doctor can be deduced from the fact that Mr Bedbrook hardly recognised him upon arrival, and that in answer to his brother-in-law's greeting: 'How fat you are looking, Percy, old boy,' the latter replied, 'I wish I could say the same of you, George.'

Mr Bedbrook then invited his guest to take a glass of sherry and this the latter accepted, but asked for some white sugar in order to neutralise the alcohol in the wine. The significance of this action is obscure, and though the point was laboured by the prosecution, it is doubtful whether this sugar played more than a subsidiary part in Lamson's scheme. The doctor had with him a bag, and from this he took a Dundee cake and some sweets. After some further conversation Lamson turned to Mr Bedbrook and remarked apropros of nothing:

'While in America, I did not forget you. I have bought these capsules for you. You will find them very useful to give the boys medicine. I should like you to try one and see how easily they can be swallowed.'

As he spoke he produced a half-empty box of capsules from the bag, gave one of them to Mr Bedbrook and then shovelling some of the sugar into another one, said: 'Here, Percy, you are a swell pill-taker; take this and show Mr Bedbrook how easily it can be swallowed.'

The boy complied, and Lamson at once said, 'I must be going now.'

Though Blenheim House was less than a minute's walk from the station, the next train left at seven twenty-one, and it was then already seven-twenty. Mr Bedbrook pointed this out to Lamson and suggested that he should go by the next train, the seven-fifty, but the other refused, declaring that he would miss the boat-train from Victoria unless he went at once. However, he stayed a minute or more saying goodbye, and it was past seven twenty-one when he left the school. It may also be noted that he succeeded in catching the boat-train, and crossed to France that night. Not knowing how soon the poison would work and distrusting his powers of dissimulation, he determined to get away before the first symptoms manifested themselves.

Twenty minutes after his departure Percy John complained of heart-burn, gradually became worse, and was carried up to bed. He was obviously suffering intense pain, and felt, he said, as he had done the previous August when Lamson had given him a pill in the Isle of Wight. He vomited frequently, and during the intervals between these attacks he was in such agony that he was with difficulty kept down by those who were holding him. Asked to describe his symptoms, he declared that his throat was closing and that his skin was being drawn up.

At five minutes to nine Dr Berry, the practitioner who regularly attended the school, arrived, and at his suggestion Dr Little, who happened to be in the house, also inspected the patient. They applied hot linseed poultices to the stomach and gave the boy white of egg beaten up in water, but without any beneficial results. Ultimately, seeing that the pain increased rather than diminished, they injected morphia at about ten o'clock. The symptoms abated somewhat as soon as the drug took effect, but shortly before eleven they returned in an even more aggravated form. A further injection produced no apparent effect, and at eleven-twenty, after four hours of the most exquisite agony, the unfortunate boy died.

That death was due to some irritant poison was the immediate, in fact, the inevitable theory of both doctors, and they at once collected a sample of the vomit in order that it might be submitted to chemical analysis. On December 6th, a post-mortem examination was held by Drs Bond, Little, and Berry, but apart from a slight congestion of one of the lungs, the body proved to be organically healthy and they could discover no natural cause of death.

Having bungled the affair at Shanklin owing to meanness, Lamson erred this time on the side of generosity, and there can be no doubt that during his visit he had succeeded in administering an exceptionally large dose of aconitine to his brother-in-law. What medium he used to convey the poison is uncertain. It was the theory of the prosecution that the fatal dose was contained in the capsule that the boy swallowed, but it will be remembered that Mr Bedbrook was standing at Lamson's elbow and saw him fill the empty shell with castor sugar. Unless the doctor added sleight of hand to his other accomplishments, it is doubtful whether poison could have been introduced into the capsule without Mr Bedbrook noticing the manœuvre.

It seems more probable that the aconitine was contained in the slice of cake which the doctor gave to Percy John, and even though the cake may not have been cut when Lamson produced it (as I have stated, there appears to be a conflict of opinion on this point), it would have been simple for him, knowing which portion he had impregnated with poison, to give that particular piece to his brother-in-law. The cake was an ordinary Dundee one, supplied by Messrs Buzzards, and all that was needed to transform it into the most certain instrument of death was to extract a few raisins near the surface, to fill them with aconitine, and to replace them, care being taken to leave some distinctive mark, so that no miscarriage of murder might arise.

If this theory is correct, and it was secretly held by counsel defending Lamson, what point could there have been in the capsule incident? That Lamson had thought out the whole performance very carefully is proved by his demand for sugar, which, in spite of his assertion, has the effect of augmenting rather than of counteracting the alcohol in sherry, and by his production of the capsules, which seem to have been bought for that special purpose and to have been introduced into the conversation apropos of nothing at all. The explanation probably is that Lamson wished to distract attention from his real plan. If suspicion of foul play arose, it would naturally be suggested that the poison had been administered in the capsule, and the fact that he had openly filled it with plain sugar right under the eyes of Mr Bedbrook must inevitably be proved in court and might go far towards establishing his plea of Not Guilty. It was an elaborate but not very skilful scheme, and though at the trial the Crown relied solely upon the capsule theory, the precise medium through which the poison was administered did not play a very cardinal part in the presentation either of the prosecution or of the defence.

Every circumstance, then, pointed to murder and to Lamson as the murderer. Who was the last person to give food to the deceased? Who would benefit financially by his death? The police had no great difficulty in reaching the obvious conclusion, and when other incidents were revealed, including the purchase of aconitine a few weeks earlier, and the elaborate lies to Tulloch, their suspicions amounted almost to certainty. Lamson's name was freely mentioned in connection with the case, and had he been in England he would have at once been detained. But he had vanished—according to his own account, to Paris, but no one could certainly say whither. Then it was that Lamson resolved upon a bold and desperate stroke; a stroke at once impudent and imprudent, yet so daring in conception that, had the case against him been less strong, it might have succeeded.

Suddenly, dramatically, he returned to London on December 8th, and going to Scotland Yard demanded to see Inspector Butcher. Questioned as to his business, he replied:

'I am Dr Lamson whose name has been mentioned in connection with the death at Wimbeldon.'

He went on to say that he had come back to clear the matter up, and he hoped that his return and his explanation would obviate any necessity of preferring an actual charge against him. After reporting his arrival to the authorities, the inspector sat chatting with him upon other topics for an hour or so, and then took him before the competent magistrate.

Lamson's nerve, which had dictated this theatrical and seemingly willing surrender, now began to desert him, and indeed afterwards he never exhibited the courage and self-control that might have been expected from so inhuman a criminal. He apparently anticipated that, owing to his voluntary return, bail would be allowed, but, as is usual in capital cases, his application was refused. And so only five days after the commission of the crime, which he had plotted probably for five months, Lamson found himself in custody, from which there could be but one deliverance, for with his education and experience he must have realised that only the miracle, which every human being half-believes will intervene in his favour, could save him from the gallows.

On March 9th, 1882, the trial opened at the Central Criminal Court before Mr Justice Hawkins. The Solicitor-General, Sir F. Herschel, led for the Crown, and with him were Mr (later Sir Harry) Poland and Mr A.L. Smith. Lamson was represented by Mr Montague Williams, Mr C. Matthews, Mr E. Gladstone, and Mr W.S. Robson.

An immense crowd had assembled outside the court, and to those who were fortunate enough to be admitted the prisoner was naturally the centre of interest. His was a face that could not easily be forgotten: a lofty forehead, a pair of dark, restless, intelligent eyes, and a thick black beard of the shape affected by Charles Dickens—in effect a lean, sinister face, but the fact of a thinker and a man of refinement. He bowed slightly to the judge, and in answer to the indictment pleaded 'Not Guilty.'

The case outlined by the Solicitor-General was an overwhelmingly strong one, and the only difficulty experienced by the prosecution was the actual proof of the presence of aconitine in the body of the deceased. At that date it was impossible to detect vegetable poisons by any chemical test, and the only analytical experiment which could be undertaken was that of tasting extracts from the various organs. Modern scientific improvements, as exemplified by the Crippen trial, have rendered more simple the process of discovering the presence of vegetable alkaloids, and one cannot but sympathise with the expert, Dr Stevenson, over what must have been an extremely unpleasant job.

Drs Little and Berry, who had attended the deceased, could give little more than a description of his death and of the results of the post-mortem examination. Both frankly confessed that they knew nothing of the properties of aconitine, and Mr Williams,w ho had been 'coached' for the case by an eminent toxicologist and was prepared to confute them with his special knowledge, had to make what capital he could out of their ignorance. It was the theory of the defence that the boy had died from pressure, caused by curvature of the spine, on the arteries, but counsel could not make the doctors commit themselves. They declined to say definitely that death could not have resulted from this cause, yet refused equally to agree that it might have done. With Mr Bond, who had assisted the local doctors at the post-mortem examination, Mr Williams had no more success. He, like the others, admitted that he was not acquainted with the various preparations of aconitia, and that he had never met a case of poisoning by that drug.

It was suggested by the defence that if aconitine was found in the body—minute traces of different poisons are frequently discovered during post-mortem examinations of people who have died from other causes—the amount was not sufficient to produce death. Here, like the preceding witnesses, Mr Bond relied upon text-books and upon personal inexperience.[1]

Mr Williams: 'Would you, supposing death had been occasioned by aconitine, expect to find the amount of poison that had caused death or would it have disappeared?—I believe it would be possible to use so small a dose that it would not be found in the stomach.' (The prisoner, after his experiment in the Isle of Wight, was probably best qualified to elucidate this point.)

'Supposing death caused by aconitine, would you expect to find the actual amount that caused death?'—'That would depend upon the amount. My opinion is that if death was caused by an ordinary amount, traces would be found.'

'Of the amount that caused death?'—'Not at all.'

The witness went on to explain that the poison would be absorbed by the other organs, but when pressed he had again to admit that he possessed no special knowledge of aconitine.

Dr Williams, therefore, had to reserve his learning for Dr Stevenson. In examination-in-chief the doctor described the various experiments that he had conducted. From the contents of the bowels he obtained, by Stass's process, an alkaloidal extract, 'which was distinctive and produced a very faint sensation like that of aconitia. When placed on the tongue, burning of the lips was produced though the extract did not touch the lips. Burning, tingling—a kind of numbness peculiar but difficult to define; a salivation creating a desire to expectorate, a sensation at the back of the throat of swelling up, and this was followed by a peculiar seared sensation of the tongue, as if a hot iron had been drawn over it.'

Later, in answer to the judge, he declared that he had between fifty and seventy alkaloids in his possession and had tasted them all. As the symptoms from this experiment with aconitine lasted acutely for over four hours, one can appreciate that Dr Stevenson's job was no sinecure.

The only other test that could be undertaken was the inoculation of mice with extracts from the organs submitted to him. In each case the injections produced precisely the same symptoms and results as an injection with Morson's Aconitia. A considerable number of mice were sacrificed in this way, and though Mr Williams in his closing speech condemned the cruelty of these experiments, there can be no doubt that they enormously strengthened the case for the prosecution.

Giving as his opinion that one-sixteeth of a grain of aconitia was a fatal dose, the witness showed how easily even a grain of the poison could be placed in a capsule; by taking it in this way, it would be impossible to detect any taste, and the burning of the tongue and lips described by Dr Stevenson would not at once occur. It may, however, be pointed out, that the same result would be achieved by filling a raisin skin with the drug.

The fact that the cake, when submitted to chemical analysis, revealed no trace of poison, does not dispose of our theory, for had aconitine been administered in the way suggested, it would not have impregnated the whole cake.

The cross-examination of Dr Stevenson was too technical to be of general interest, but though it proved the profound study that Mr Williams had devoted to the case, it failed to shake either the authority of the witness or the strength of the case for the prosecution. It was an ordeal from which few would have emerged with so much credit.

With witness as to fact, such as Mr Bedbrook and Mr Tulloch, counsel was slightly more successful. Under the questioning of so skilled an advocate they were made to contradict themselves over non-essential matters, yet the main outline of the story remained untouched and damning. One rather curious piece of testimony was the evidence given by the assistants of Messrs Allen and Hanbury's, where it was alleged Lamson had purchased aconitine. On hearing that Lamson's name had been mentioned in connection with the death of Percy John, they recalled that he had visited their shop. Looking up their note of the sale, they came to the conclusion that the drug which he had bought was atrophine, which is also a vegetable poison.

Later, before there had been any suggestion that aconitine had been discovered in the body of the deceased, they changed their opinion, on account of the price of the drug, and informed the police that the doctor had bought from them two grains of aconitine. Oddly enough, Lamson had been in the habit of mixing atrophine with morphia for the self-injections in which he indulged, but thought Mr Williams pointed out the probability that atrophine, not aconitine, had been purchased, the witnesses refused to accept his correction.

For the defence no evidence was called. The Criminal Evidence Act had not then been passed, and the prisoner was not, therefore, a competent witness; while, apparently, everyone else who could in any way testify to the facts of the case had already been placed in the box by the prosecution.

Mr Williams was therefore unable to urge the probability of any opposing story, and had to content himself with demonstrating the improbability of the story presented by the Crown. His speech lasted for many hours, and though here and there rather florid and rhetorical, it must rank as one of the most eloquent and moving appeals ever heard in a criminal court—an example of the old school of oratory which is now fast disappearing. But it was a gallant effort in a hopeless cause. The facts themselves stood out stark and incontrovertible, and though he could disguise them beneath ingenious explanations he was unable to do more than confuse some of the minor issues. He waxed indignant over Dr Stevenson's treatment of mice; he discovered a scandal in the refusal of the authorities to allow Lamson to be represented at the chemical analysis; he drew a pathetic picture of the prisoner's devoted wife, who if the jury's verdict was adverse, would be condemned to worse than death.

This was all very fine, but the Solicitor-General's unemotional reply, which pointed out that the facts prosecuted by the Crown had not seriously been challenged, nullified its effect, and by the time Sir Henry Hawkins had finished his dispassionate review of the evidence, Mr William's sentimental thunder was almost forgotten. After an absence of three-quarters of an hour the jury returned a verdict of Guilty, and Lamson, 'protesting his innocence before God,' was sentenced to death.

Strenuous efforts to save him were now made by friends both in England and America, and the fact that they should have rallied round him in this crisis proves that there must have been something likeable about the man. That so charming a companion could commit so appalling a crime argued insanity. Affidavits, covering a number of years, were filed to show that Lamson's brain had for a long time been abnormal, and that his addiction to the morphine habit had destroyed his ethical sense and left him defenceless against his homicidal impulse.

One of the most illuminating of these documents was sworn by a comrade of Lamson's who had served with him at Bukarest during the Balkan War of 1877. Whilst there 'he exhibited a mania for the administration of aconitine in almost every case, using it in season and out of season, and in such quantities as to alarm the medical staff and to render his recall to England necessary.' Another affidavit dealt with his conduct at the siege of Paris in 1871, where his reckless use of drugs made him a public danger; while from America came a declaration signed by three eminent doctors, who had met him the previous summer (1881) to the effect that morphine injections had undoubtedly turned his brain. 'He passed the greater part of the day either dozing or attempting to read. He was then using a mixture apparently of morphia and atropine, but said that he preferred aconitine but could not procure it in that section of the country.' Dr Winston, the medical director of the New York Mutual Life Assurance Company, considered 'that he had become a helpless victim of the habit, which had seriously impaired his mental powers and destroyed his moral responsibility;' Mr Murrary declared 'that he was utterly irresponsible for his acts.'

Other evidence tried to prove that he was tainted with hereditary insanity from the fact that his grandmother had been an inmate of the New York Bloomingdale Asylum, but as she was not removed there until the age of seventy-six, this was not a very cogent piece of testimony.

Lastly, his solicitor deposed that 'he could obtain no assistance from him in the preparation of his defence—that he appeared to have no memory and to be incapable of appreciating the bearing of any of the facts of his case or the gravity of his position!'

In deference to this universal clamour, the Home Secretary, Sir William Harcourt, postponed the date of the execution in order that these affidavits might be considered, and a further respite was granted at the request of President Arthur to allow the documents from America to reach their destination. But after perusing them Sir William found himself unable to recommend the Queen to exercise her prerogative of mercy; nor can there be any doubt that he was right. The defence of insanity had not been raised at the trial, and even had it been urged with all the eloquence at Mr Williams' command, it is inconceivable that the jury would have returned a different verdict. The burden of proving insanity rests, of course, upon the defence, and, as I have already pointed out, it must be established that the state of the prisoner's mind was such that he could not realise the nature and quality of his acts. How could this be said of Lamson, who must have appreciated the pecuniary benefit he would derive from the death of Percy John? Or, if it be suggested that the crime was the result of homicidal mania, why should he have selected this victim? The motive for the murder was too convincing to support a plea of insanity.

The execution was ultimately fixed for April 28th, nearly six weeks after the conviction, and the well-meant efforts of his friends to win a reprieve served only to aggravate the prisoner's anguish. Fear rather than remorse dominated him, and his mental agony must have been in proportion to the physical suffering he had inflicted upon his victim. Courage and comfort he could find only in the morphia needle, and the reaction, resulting from his inability to secure the drug in prison, completely prostrated him. One moment he seemed oblivious of what awaited him, the next, knowledge returned with redoubled terror.

A few days before his execution he wrote a long rambling document, which appears to be an admission of his guilt, and he also made a verbal confession to the chaplain; but he denied upon oath that he was in any way responsible for the death of Herbert John, and it may be that the world, loath to believe that any murderer is ever hanged for his first murder, is in this instance mistaken. It was not to be expected that he would meet his end with the fortitude that goes some way towards redeeming the memory of his peers. Here was no stoic, but a poor, weak soul, appalled beyond conception at the prospect of death. Realising upon that fatal morning that his time had come, he abandoned all effort at composure and was helped, almost unconscious, to the scaffold. There, unable to stand, he was held upon the drop by two warders, and even as the hangman was pulling the lever, he tried to snatch another minute of life by begging the chaplain to recite just one more prayer.

Had he been tried to-day, when so much more is known about abnormality, he might have escaped the consequence of his crime. Of the fact that he was not altogether normal there is abundant evidence; but who has a brain so nice that it can apportion responsibility between morphia, poverty, desperation, and chance?

LEONARD GRIBBLE
The Long Island Borgia

The man who had received the three poison-pen letters had come to a reluctant decision. The flow of vituperation must be stopped, and there was only one way he could do that. He took the letters to the office of the local district attorney, Martin W. Littleton, who was not in when he called. This left him rather nonplussed. The one calculation he had not made was what to do if he didn't see the district attorney. Instead of leaving that office in Mineola, Long Island, he decided to unburden himself to Martin Littleton's assistant, a young man of less experience.

He was shown into the younger man's office, and introduced himself as Everett Applegate, who was an official in the American Legion in Nassau County.

'I'd like you to look at this stuff that's been sent to me,' he said. 'I want to know what you can do to stop it.' He pushed three letters on to the assistant district attorney's desk. 'Something must be done,' he insisted.

Each of the envelopes bore the same inscription: 'To the People at 12 Bryant Place, Baldwin, Long Island,' and contained a sheet of yellow paper torn from a pad of lined writing paper which was covered with identical writing. The messages were all couched in similar terms. A typical one charged:

'I know I speak for your neighbours when I tell you that we are sick and tired of two people living on this street. You don't need to guess that I could only mean Everett Applegate and that fat Ada, his wife. Applegate is no good and never was. He is a wolf in sheep's clothing and is on the make for every woman he meets. As for his wife, she has a mouth as big as she is. She uses it to tell lies about the people she lives with and they are foolish to let her pull the wool over their eyes that way.'

The three letters had been posted on consecutive days, the last on 19

June, 1935, a Wednesday. Everett Applegate was making his protest on the Friday.

The frowning young lawyer behind the desk read them through, looked at the envelopes, and asked who had received them. His visitor explained that he and his wife and daughter lodged with a husband and wife named Creighton. Mrs Creighton had received the post and handed the letters to her lodger. The Creightons had a son and daughter. Asked if he had any idea who could have sent the anonymous letters the caller said that was his predicament. He had no idea who would have written them, but he wanted them stopped.

The lawyer's frown did not lift as he explained that none of the letters was obscene. They were objectionable and cowardly, but their terms were not such that the district attorey's office could take direct action against the person who had written them. However, he kept the letters for reference. His caller, disappointed and frustrated, left, but did not return with any further letters written in similar terms. Three months passed. The poison-pen letters had been forgotten when suddenly Mrs Applegate died.

That sudden death apparently interested a neighbour in Baldwin who had a good memory. She went to the local public library and waded through back numbers until she found a report of what was described as a murder in New Jersey. It had happened a dozen years before. The Creightons had been arrested for poisoning Mrs Creighton's brother Raymond Avery with arsenic. The motive was claimed to be a sum in insurance that would be paid on Raymond Avery's death. However, the evidence was not sufficiently strong to implicate the accused, and the jury hearing the case decided that murder had not been proved. The Creightons were acquitted of the charge against them and freed.

The woman with the memory of court case details was Mrs Olive Salket. Having searched the newspaper records for the past twelve years and found what she had remembered, she had a photostatic copy of the evidence taken, which she sent to the police, who upon inquiry learned that Mrs Salket had once accused Mrs Creighton of stealing money from her handbag on an occasion when she visited the other woman's home. The quarrel had been patched up when Mrs Creighton explained that she could not have been responsible. But it was at best an uneasy truce between neighbours with no great fondness for each other. However, in order, as she claimed, to make things right between them Mrs Creighton a short while after the quarrel brought Mrs Salket a cake.

'I baked it myself, and it's a peace offering,' she smiled, 'so please accept it in the spirit in which I offer it.'

The cake had been accepted and Mrs Creighton thanked. But when later she ate a slice of the home-made cake Mrs Salket became violently ill and was sick. It took her several days to recover, and when she had she called on Mrs Creighton and told her what had happened.

'I believe you deliberately tried to poison me,' she accused.

Instead of being intimidated or confused by such blunt words Mary Creighton laughed.

'Go around repeating that, Olive,' she said, 'and I promise you'll be sorry. I'll claim damages for malicious slander. Years back someone tried that in New Jersey, and I made them very sorry. Very sorry indeed.'

It was the reference to New Jersey that had provided the clue on which Olive Salket acted with considerable diligence. Now the police had something on which to act, both a complaint and some evidence. They sought out Everett Applegate, the lodger who had lost his amply proportioned wife.

He was asked what he knew about his landlord and wife. At the same time the police made routine inquiries about Ada Applegate's sudden death. For his part Everett Applegate spoke freely about the Creightons. He explained that he knew all about their arrest in Newark, New Jersey and the trial at which they had been acquitted on what Mary Creighton had insisted was a frame-up.

'They're nice people,' he told the police. 'They were kind to my wife, who was ill for about a year before she died.'

'So her death wasn't really sudden?' a detective asked.

'I wasn't expecting it. Let me put it like that. After all, Ada had been ill for a long time, but I didn't suspect it was as serious as it turned out to be.' He shook his head, as though puzzled by something. 'What she actually died of was trouble with her gall bladder, and the complications that condition set up.'

The physician who had attended her lived in a nearby neighbourhood known as Malverne. He had signed the death certificate within a short time of her death. To be sure of what they were inquiring into, the police asked the district attorney's office if there was any reference on their files to either the Creightons or the Applegates. That was when the poison-pen letters were taken from the file where they had been collecting summer dust. Inspector H.R. King, in charge of Nassau County's detective division, read through the letters and found them odd. As he told a colleague, 'In the circumstances I would have expected the writer to have been Mrs Salket, except that the writer's attack is directed at the lodgers, not the Creightons. So something appears to be wrong, which lets out Mrs Salket.'

Worried by what seemed to him a discrepancy, he visited the Malverne doctor, who confessed that he too had a worry and admitted that he signed Mrs Applegate's death certificate against his better judgment, because he had been for some time treating her for one complaint, but she had died of another.

'In such circumstances I normally insist on an autopsy as a matter of course, but I was persuaded against that because I was told it would mean much talk in the district.'

In answer to questions he explained that he had been treating the woman of thirty-six, who weighed nearly twenty stone, for obesity for a year, and had been suddenly summoned to her bedside to find her suffering from nausea and sickness.

'I had her sent to hospital, and curiously while there her condition improved, but she had not been home five hours, undergoing an identical treatment, when the nausea and vomiting returned.'

When her husband phoned him to come quickly he found his patient dead, and could only decide that coronary occlusion was the immediate cause of death. The doctor also told the detective chief that Mrs Creighton had been very concerned about his patient and had usually been in attendance when he called at Bryant Place. When asked if he considered arsenic might have induced the nausea and vomiting he was plainly shocked, because the implications were only too plain, but he was forced to agree that such symptoms as he had found were consistent with arsenical poisoning.

As a result of this visit to Malverne the three adults at 12 Bryant Place were, at the request of the district attorney, taken to police headquarters. Everett Applegate seemed voluble and distracted by the enforced visit, which was made late at night. But John Creighton and his wife Mary had little to say. The former was a quiet, unassuming man who appeared puzzled by the police interest. Mary, a Junoesque figure of a dark-eyed woman with brown hair, who appeared to be in her late thirties, smiled but kept her mouth shut. Her glance was directed at the face of Martin W. Littleton, the district attorney Everett Applegate had not seen when he called with the poison-pen letters.

Now Martin Littleton had much more than three spite-filled letters on his legal plate. What he wanted to do was establish if the circumst-ances and conditions of Raymond Avery's death in New Jersey had borne any resemblance to those of Ada Applegate's on Long Island.

John Creighton, who worked in the county engineer's office in Mineola, didn't seem to get the drift of the interrogation. He kept shaking his puzzled head. But not Mary Creighton. She readily admit-ted the similarity of conditions and circumstances, but claimed to have pointed this out to the doctor, who told her that there were several type of illness that produced regular bouts of nausea and vomiting.

'So I thought it was natural.'

She even smiled when she said it, though the sharp eyes watching her could not perceive any amusement in the smile. Mary Frances Creight-on just looked confident as though she was telling the truth and so knew she had nothing to fear.

District Attorney Littleton wondered. He had met many kinds of women. Mary Creighton seemed to be in a category of her own. It was as though she was compulsively good-natured, which he strongly sus-pected.

But he felt that something was compelling her to behave in the way she was.

She told him that she and Everett Applegate, between them, prepared the sick woman's meals. She was switched to talk about Olive Salket, but admitted that she did not get on with the other woman.

'I don't know why she is like she is towards me, unless it was that cake I gave her. But then I've never pretended to be any good at cake-mixing. They never turn out to be to my liking. For instance, they never rise properly. They always sag.'

Turning back to Applegate, the district attorney was told that they all lived in a very small house with only two bedrooms on the ground floor and other bedrooms that were makeshift places, even the back porch being turned into one for the Creightons' son.

'The idea was to share expenses,' Applegate confided.

The Creightons confirmed this, even admitted having occasional overnight guests who were squeezed in somewhere when they 'doubled up'. On one such occasion a Creighton female board of fifteen shared the room with the adult Applegates.

'Why not your own daughter?' Everett Applegate was asked.

'Because we liked the kid. Evelyn's like another daughter to me.'

However, Martin Littleton could not but feel that too many things about this household were unusual. He pushed a form forward for Applegate to sign.

'Why?' asked the man offered a pen. 'What's it for?'

'It's your authority for us to exhume Mrs Applegate's body so that we may have an autopsy.'

Applegate twirled the pen around in his fingers for some moments of indecision, but he realized he was backed up with no chance of refusing. He signed his name where instructed.

Before they left the Creightons were asked to make detailed statements about the dead woman's last hours. They offered no objection. But later, after the statements signed by the Creightons were gone over it was discovered that, when they were compared with Everett Applegate's anonymous poison-pen letters, the person who had written the latter had also written and signed one of the new statements—Mary Creighton.

This time Mary Creighton was interviewed alone. She was accused of having written the letters on the lined yellow pages torn from a cheap pad. She was not a bit flustered by such a confrontation. She kept her smile in place, and shrugged her wide shoulders as she adjusted the hat on her dark hair.

'You know, I never could disguise anything,' she said. 'It isn't in my nature.'

She even sounded complacent.

'But why did you write them and send them to your own home?' she was asked.

'Oh, that's simple,' she said, finding some more dimples in her wide cheeks. 'I wanted the Applegates out of the house and gone. I'd had enough of them. I didn't like to ask John to tell them to go. He's soft about people. Too kind-hearted. I thought it would be best to do it this way.'

She was asked if there wasn't some other reason.

'Since you put it like that, yes. Everett is a bad influence around a house with young girls,' giving the impression that the opinion was being dragged from her reluctantly. 'Besides, he was always making passes at me.'

Mary Creighton was allowed to join her husband and Applegate. By this time Dr Carl Hettescheimer, who was medical examiner for Nassau County, had received the necessary authority to open Mrs Applegate's grave, remove her body and perform a post-mortem. This was done in the middle of the night while the examination of the three adults continued. Suddenly the district attorney's phone rang.

It was the medical examiner with a preliminary report. He had found the dead woman's kidneys swollen excessively and her liver noticeably inflamed.

'This is consistent with poisoning by arsenic,' he told Martin Littleton, who now felt he had plenty to justify his night without sleep. Within a few hours he would receive the medical examiner's formal analysis of the stomach and other organs.

He returned to Mary Creighton. Her smile wasn't so fresh, but it was still in evidence. She admitted that she had not been afraid of Everett Applegate.

'But I didn't want to upset John by telling him about Everett's making passes at me. He would have been very upset, and I wanted to avoid that for his sake. That's why I wrote those letters, like I told you. I wanted to get the Applegates out of the house. I thought those letters would do it.'

'Were you surprised when they didn't?' she was asked.

'I was disappointed. But then I've thought since that it was probably foolish to send them. I'm not good at writing.'

That made two things she was not good at, the district attorney recalled. The other was baking a cake. He decided she should be interviewed by a psychiatrist, and it was a short time later that a well-known psychiatrist from New York, Dr Richard Hoffman, arrived on Long Island in reply to a telephone call.

He was told an outline of the case and requested to go to Bryant Place and interview the occupants against their own background.

'I'd like a special report on the girl Evelyn, who is only fifteen,' said Littleton.

Dr Hoffman certainly found the household he visited more unique than usual. But the girl Evelyn was an assured and self-contained minor who called Everett Applegate Uncle Ev. However, although she was assured that she need not feel embarrassed in answering the psychiatrist's questions, she coloured brightly when she answered truthfully about her intimate relationship with Uncle Ev, which had continued since the previous June, just before the anonymous letters arrived.

Mary Creighton was asked if she had been aware of the relations between her young boarder and Applegate. She appeared horrified.

'Certainly not,' she asserted.

But the girl claimed Mrs Creighton had known about it from the beginning. 'She caught us in bed,' she told Dr Hoffman.

'Did Mrs Applegate know?'

'Sure, and Aunt Ada was mad, but not at me—at Uncle Ev.'

According to the girl Applegate had frequently told her he loved her and wanted to marry her. The house was searched but the police found nothing to interest them, and at a conference with the district attorney the question was raised why Mary Creighton didn't have Applegate charged with statutory rape for having sexual intercourse with a minor.

'There can only be one answer to why she sent those letters and didn't charge him with rape,' said Inspector King. 'Applegate has something on her.'

The decision was taken to keep all members of the house at 12 Bryant Place closely watched until the New York analyst's report on Ada Applegate's post-mortem was received. Meantime the New Jersey cases were studied and produced a surprise. Mary Creighton had been charged with murder not just once, but twice, and been acquitted. Not long after being acquitted of poisoning Raymond Avery, her brother, the woman was charged with similarly poisoning her mother-in-law, Mrs Walter Creighton. Again a jury acquitted her, and in both instances she secured a sizeable sum in insurance.

It seemed success in the past had become a compulsive habit. A week after receiving Mrs Salket's photostats, on 5 October, a report was received from New York. Enough arsenic had been found in Ada Applegate's stomach to kill four persons. The district attorney took the findings to Bryant Place and surprised Mary Creighton by asking her how long she had been having sexual relations with the dead woman's husband.

'Not since he started with Evelyn,' she snapped. 'Before that he blackmailed me about the New Jersey trials, which I didn't want our boy to know about.'

She also said Ada Applegate had what she called a mean mouth and was bent on making trouble for her. In effect it meant that Mary Creighton and Everett Applegate both wanted to be rid of the fat wife. She was accused of poisoning Ada Applegate's food, but she insisted Everett was in the plot to sprinkle patent vermin killer called 'Rough On Rats' in the doomed woman's food.

Once she had made this admission it was as though she had only one idea, to involve Applegate. She had told him, she claimed, that he could get a tin of 'Rough On Rats' from any drugstore without having to sign it.

'I told him I'd used it on my brother and mother-in-law,' she said, keen to be believed. 'He told me he'd get it if he thought we could really use it without being found out. That's when I told him I'd used it successfully twice before.'

According to this middle-aged woman whose success as a poisoner had gone to her head, she had still to convince her confederate, but at last Everett Applegate's fears were resolved.

'We'll get the stuff together,' he decided, and she couldn't see why it should take two of them, but agreed with him.

Even so, when they took a car to a chemist's in Merrick Road, it was she who had to get out and go into the shop and buy the patent paste for exterminating rodents. She paid twenty-three cents for the box, which contained a greyish compound of arsenic mixed with lamp black.

'It's not only rough on rats,' she said, smiling as she showed it to the man waiting for her and settled herself into the seat beside him.

Later that day, when preparing the food for the sick Ada Applegate, Mary Creighton decided to make a chocolate pudding, which she knew was a favourite dessert of the woman she was about to poison.

'But of course I had to make sure that no one else in the house ate any,' she told her listeners.

By this time it was as though she was enjoying making a full confession so that the persons watching her would be able to appreciate how smart she had been, particularly at making sure Everett Applegate, who had turned to a teenager in preference to herself and her own appeal, was involved so that he would not be able to extricate himself from the guilt she was piling on him. And of course then he would not be in a position to marry Evelyn.

Behind her smile and dark eyes Mary Creighton was a devious woman. She wanted a new success which was sudeenly important to her. To make sure Applegate, the timid man with inconsistent moods, was branded as a murderer.

'Rough On Rats' was not only mixed into the chocolate pudding served to Ada Applegate, it was also whipped into culinary gravies and some sauces specially prepared for the doomed invalid. One thing was sure. Mary Creighton was clever at disguising an unpleasant taste, except in the case of Olive Salket. In this she was not unique. She had her counterpart in most countries that have a long record of criminal violence and police investigation. But she was compelled by former success to try murder as en encore in precisely the same manner with which she had previously been successful. It was those former successes that encouraged her and became compulsive as a driving force to motive.

Her explanation revealed, of course, why Ada Applegate had recovered during her visit to hospital and why she had a return of her former nausea and vomiting as soon as she returned to the house in Bryant Place.

Indeed, her return to the small house where her death had been assured was callously celebrated by a special glass of egg nog, for which she had a special yearning.

'And I'll make you one of your favourite chocolate puddings,' promised the woman doing everything she could to repeat success for the third time.

26 September, 1935, was a Thursday. The intended victim's death loomed on the horizon of her remaining hours of life. She had been virtually stuffed with soft and liquid foods that had been potently mixed with 'Rough On Rats'. Without her doctor being aware of the fact, her resistance had become so low through her arsenical intake that recovery was virtually impossible.

Indeed, it was on that day that Ada Applegate could be said to have reached the lethal point of no return. She could only continue to her death.

In his own statement the now fully inculpated Everett Applegate did the expected turn-about and rounded on his former mistress. According to him Mary Creighton took him on one side in the kitchen and said sharply, 'Come on, let's stop fooling around and mix a good strong dose. I'm getting tired of waiting for it to be over and done with.'

The reason for this show of impatience, according to her confederate in crime, was that Ada Applegate's appetite for food was failing rapidly by this time.

'I can't take any more, Mary,' she kept saying pitifully.

But Mary Creighton, the smiling false friend, insisted that she had prepared a fresh egg nog specially for the invalid.

'It'll give you strength, dear. Here, leh me hold your head up. That'll make it easier.'

So Ada Applegate was virtually force-fed the lethal dose that drained away the last of her life.

Mary Creighton was convinced that, for the third time, success had attended her murderous experiments with 'Rough on Rats', and when

Everett Applegate talked his dead wife's surprised doctor into making out a death certificate in order to avoid the possibility of gossip and scandal throughout the neighbourhood she was also convinced that she had got away with murder for the third time in a row.

As she very well might have done if she hadn't given that sick-making and poorly baked cake to Olive Salket, who proved in the event to be an unusual harbinger of retribution, prepared to spend hours at a public library digging up the records of a murder trial of a dozen years before in Newark, New Jersey. But as has been pointed out a great many times, justice often moves in a mysterious way.

The female poisoner who now had nothing to smile at or for was asked, as a point of routine, if she had put any of her notorious 'Rough on Rats' in the cake she had baked and given to Mrs Salket.

'Perhaps just a pinch or two,' was all she would admit, and justified it in her own eyes by claiming that Olvie Salket shouldn't have accused her of taking a few dollars from her handbag. 'She had it coming to her,' were her final words on the subject of what might have been another poisoning murder.

When it came time for Everett Applegate to make his own detailed statement, he too had a surprise and even a shock for the police and district attorney's officers who heard him. With fairly cool detachment he admitted to being involved in poisoning his wife, but insisted that the actual feeding of the poisoned food was done by Mary Creighton. What he most strongly insisted was that the woman who had used 'Rough On Rats' with such inhuman optimism had never been his mistress. Somehow this subject brought out every stubborn objection in his nature.

'She was too old for me. I couldn't bring myself to have sex with her. The very idea was repulsive.'

Was this merely a curious and very personal tit for tat by a man who had only one way that he saw of showing his contempt for the accomplice who had deliberately involved him in a crime both must answer for?

It is at least possible. Perhaps he had hoped to share in Mary Creighton's continued murder success story, only to discover when too late that third time could be unlucky. Or had those anonymous poison-pen letters festered for too long in his mind, breeding a different kind of poison?

That too was possible.

The trial did not resolve these points. It opened on Thursday, 15 January, 1936, at Mineola, with Judge Courtland A. Johnson on the

Bench. The defendants were the pair who had together worked to bring about the death of Ada Applegate. The husband's defence was a bland denial of poisoning his wife. He claimed that if his wife was poisoned, then Mary Creighton must have fed the poison to her. Mary Creighton had also undergone a change of mind if not precisely of that stone which she considered her heart. She insisted her alleged confession was a tissue of lies that had been tricked out of her, but she went one better. She described Everett Applegate as mixing that last large dose of the arsenical poison in his wife's egg nog.

'You knew the arsenic came from a tin of 'Rough On Rats'?' she was asked.

She nodded and said quietly, 'Yes'.

The judge interrupted to ask her if she realized the importance of such an admission.

'Yes,' she repeated.

That pratically ended the hearing that had taken a little longer than a week. Both defendants were found guilty of murder in the first degree by a jury that did not take over-long to reach their verdict, and Judge Johnson delivered the death sentence prescribed by law. The pair were to die in the electric chair at Sing Sing. It was 25 January.

Nearly six months were taken up with a series of appeals that did not change the verdict, for they all failed. Execution was set for 16 July, 1936, by which time Mary Creighton was learning the cruelty that sometimes accompanies success, for her mind was sick with fear. Everett Applegate walked to the green-painted electric chair, but Mary Creighton was unable to move her limbs. It was as though paralysis had overtaken her.

She was almost unconscious when the woman the newspapers had labelled the 'Long Island Borgia' was lifted into a wheelchair and trundled towards that room where death awaited her when a switch was pulled.

Whatever Mary Creighton had done in her life, she can only be said to have made a very poor exit from it.

MORRIS MARKEY
The Case of the Poisoned Bun

It was during that spell of vicious heat, a little time ago, and it can hardly be doubted that the dreadful weight of air in the streets had something to do with Jellinek's final decision. But he was at the end of his tether anyway. He had to have a hundred dollars and he could think of no way at all to find it. So he went into a drug store and bought forty-five cents' worth of powdered cyanide.

When you read the simple facts, it always seems absurd that the want of a mere hundred dollars can make life unendurable. Then you may think about it a little and understand that there is a bleak reality about a hundred dollars. About ten dollars. It is the need of a million which turns out to be fantastic and even a trifle ludicrous.

Jellinek was fifty years old and he had a one-man garage business on Tenth Avenue. The creditors were snapping behind him like dogs at the heels of a tired mule. There were no customers to speak of. The heat flowed in waves along the sidewalk. Instead of going on and opening up the garage for another day, he went into the drug store and told the clerk what he wanted.

Now you see a woman named Lillian Rosenfeld—a ragamuffin woman with a soiled face—creeping out of the cellar where she lives. She walks along the street while Jellinek is in the drug store. She has never heard of Jellinek or his hundred dollars.

He came on out of the drug store and stood watching the traffic for a little while. I do not suppose he was thinking very much about anything. He just stood there for a time with his fingers around the package in his coat pocket. Then, when the light changed, he wandered across the street and through the doors of the Automat. This was the Automat at Broadway and 104th Street. It was just a few minutes before nine o'clock.

Lillian Rosenfeld, creeping along the sidewalk in her rags, decides to drop into the Automat and see if there is any business to be done. Her particular sort of business.

Jellinek had some silver left in his pocket. He changed a dime into two nickels, and went up to that fabulous dovecote where the holes are shut with thick glass. He peered through the glass and decided on two buns—two long rolls with poppy seeds upon them. He put one of his nickels into the slot, and the thick glass door popped free, and the rolls belonged to him. He walked slowly over to one of the white-topped tables, a vacant one, and sat for a considerable time looking at the two rolls.

Through the doorway comes Lillian Rosenfeld. She moves slowly, darting her eyes this way and that among the confusion of people who bend over their plates, silently swallowing their breakfasts. She fumbles the empty paper bag she holds in her hand, creeps at last toward a corner where she can be among the shadows and see everything with her birdlike eyes. Jellinek does not glance toward her. His thoughts are upon affairs more grave than ragged women who drift in from the streets.

He did not write a note. He had nothing to say, or perhaps he weighed and at last dismissed the notion of setting his unsteady thoughts upon a scrap of paper. Among all those people, urgently feeding their bellies against another wearing day, the ultimate loneliness had already begun to fall about him. Already, the workaday world with its workaday inhabitants had grown a trifle remote and inconsequential.

His hand came out of his pocket. The fingers of both hands worked at opening the small package. Presently it lay open before him, in its middle a spoonful of white powder, heaped into a little mound. The powder was ground fine, and you might have thought it was sugar—the sort they sprinkle upon pastries.

Jellinek selected one of the rolls, and pinch by pinch he dropped the powder over it, spreading the white powder among the poppy seeds until the roll was thickly covered. He did it very neatly, using all of the powder and crumpling the paper in which it had been wrapped, putting the paper in a little ball back into his pocket. Then he took a bite of the roll and swallowed it down as quickly as he could.

Almost at once he felt the shock of illness.

It would appear that those fragments of manners which had survived from his childhood surged automatically now into his fading mind. There must not be a scene. It would not be nice to upset all those people sitting quietly at breakfast. He would go off somewhere alone.

So he got up and found his way down the steps into the basement.

Now, indeed, the stars of Henry Jellinek, 605 West 170th Street, and of Lillian Rosenfeld, 119 West 104th Street, swung together in whatever cosmic pasture they were gambolling, and collided.

She had moved to the mezzanine the better to look down upon the trivial happenings about the tables. And as he got up and went away, she saw business. Her kind of business. She was up like a hawk. Like a hawk she swooped toward the table he had left. Her fingers picked up, first, the whole untouched bun and popped it into her paper bag. Then she grasped the half-eaten bun with the white powder spread among its poppy seeds, and went back to her perch, and munched the bun until it was all consumed.

It did not take the ambulance more than ten minutes to get there after she had toppled from her chair to the floor and the boy who gathers up the empty trays had gone running to the manager, urging him to telephone.

The doctor examined her and saw that she was very badly off. He told his men to carry her to the ambulance, and they were lifting her to the stretcher when a man came hurrying. There was, the man said, somebody lying on the floor in the basement, not far from the washroom door.

The doctor went down to see. Jellinek muttered something as the doctor bent over him, and then he died. Lillian Rosenfeld died just after they got her into a bed at the hospital.

You can understand well enough why the police thought, at first, that it was a double suicide. But later, when they had time to look into the odd circumstance of two people dying at nearly the same time, of cyanide sprinkled upon the same roll, they knew how it happened.

The riddle was not hard to solve after they had visited the cellar room where Lillian Rosenfeld had lived.

It was a magpie's nest. For thirty years she had spent every waking moment prowling and plucking, nipping up from the gutters and the streets and the rubbish heaps of the town an incredible store of things thrown away and things lost.

Her cellar room, two flights down, was stuffed to the ceiling with pasteboard boxes—hundreds and hundreds of pasteboard boxes which bulged with bits of rag, and string, and leather, with old shoes and old bottles and worn-out things of metal. On the floor was an inch-deep drift of peanut hulls and paper wrappings from penny sticks of chewing gum. The piles of useless junk shut out the light and air that might have found their way through the half-window, and in one corner was a tumbling bedstead, without a mattress.

The janitor of the building said that he had always felt sorry for her, seeing that she was a woman nearly fifty and that prowling through rubbish heaps was a thin way to make a living at best. Once or twice he had been sympathetic when she made excuses for not paying the seven dollars that was her monthly rent.

Listening to him, the police knew what had happened. They had learned already that she could not possibly have known Jellinek. She had gone into the Automat in the hope of finding a few left-over crumbs on somebody's plate. The whole bun and the half-bun left behind by Jellinek had been a marvellous windfall—until the poison clutched her.

'A chiseler,' the police said. 'Probably hasn't spent a penny on food in ten years—any penny at all except that seven bucks a month.'

Then they searched a while longer among a pile of filthy bedding, and found six bankbooks. It seemed that her father, dying many years ago, bequeathed a little fortune to her, and there was the customary accumulation of interest. The full amount of the deposits listed in the bankbooks was $45,000.

Jellinek needed his hundred so desperately that morning.

W.H. WILLIAMSON
Madeleine Smith

Passion is unpredictable. No one can tell where it will lead.

Pierre Emile l'Angelier was described as a 'respectable' person in 1854. He was a clerk in the firm of Huggins & Co., merchants, of Glasgow. At that time he was acquainted with a youth, Robert Baird, seventeen years of age, whose family knew some people living in India Street, Glasgow, called Smith.

Madeleine Hamilton Smith was the eldest daughter. Her father was an architect of good social standing in the city, and when Emile l'Angelier saw Madeleine Smith she had just left boarding school and was about nineteen.

We don't know very much about L'Angelier, but we have glimpses of him working hard and pursuing women like a Frenchman. To quote from the speech of the Dean of the Faculty, 'He was an unknown adventurer; utterly unknown at that time, so far as we can see. For how he procured his introduction into the employment of Huggins & Co. does not appear; and even the persons, who knew him there, knew nothing of his history or antecedents. . . . We find he is a native of Jersey; and we have discovered that at a very early period of his life, in the year 1843, he was in Scotland; he was known for three years at that time to one of the witnesses as being in Edinburgh, and the impression which he made as a very young man, which he then was, was certainly, to say the least of it, not of a very favourable kind. He goes to the Continent; he is there during the French Revolution, and he returns to this country, and is found in Edinburgh again in the year 1851. And in what condition is he then? In great poverty, in deep dejection, living upon the bounty of a tavern keeper, associating and sleeping in the same bed with the waiter of that establishment. He goes from Edinburgh to Dundee, and we trace his history there; at length we find him in Glasgow in 1853. In considering the character and conduct of the individual, whose history it is impossible to dissociate from this inquiry, we are bound to form as just an estimate as we can of what his qualities were, of what his character was, of what were the principles and motives that were likely to influence his conduct. We find him, according to the confession of all those who observed him then most narrowly, vain, conceited, pretentious, with a great opinion of his own personal attractions and a very silly expectation of admiration from the other sex. That he was to a certain extent successful in attracting such admiration may be a fact; but, at all events, his own prevailing idea seems to have been that he was calculated to be very successful in paying attentions to ladies, and that he was looking to push his fortune by that means. And accordingly once and again we find him engaged in attempts to get married to women of some station at least in society; we have heard of one disappointment which he met with in England, and another we heard a good deal of connected with a lady in the county of Fife; and the manner in which he bore his disappointment on those two occasions is perhaps the best indication and light we have as to the true character of the man. He was depressed and melancholy beyond description; he threatened—whether he intended or not—to commit suicide in consequence of his disappointment. . . .'

The Dean of the Faculty, in making those remarks, was desirous of removing sympathy from Emile L'Angelier. They seem to go a little too far when the man's hard life is pointed out as if in scorn. There is credit in rising from the half-bed of the tavern keeper. Even Robert Bruce had his moments of disappointment, and many a Scotsman could point with pride to a humble cot. 'Honour and shame from no condition rise.' But the rest of the picture gives us something of the mercurial woman chaser. There is no need for us to slander the dead: Emile L'Angelier was attracted by women. He was attracted by this girl, who had left boarding school and, whether his motives were social advancement or mere sexual urge, he was determined to know Madeleine Smith.

He got to know her.

One is inclined to think of their first meetings. The girl, brought up in a well-to-do, but probably strict, Glasgow home, meets a Frenchman. . . . To her at that moment a good deal of the romance of her silent hours is flowering. . . . He is experienced. He sees the glow in her eyes, the enchantment of her parted lips, and talks with just that ease and fire and desire to captivate, that the Frenchman can summon up for these pursuing occasions. Others too, of course.

The acquaintance ripens. She must have been thrilled by these early meetings. They were all clandestine, for she dared not tell her father. Then she had qualms. Perhaps she feared discovery and thought the best way to end the business. But it is easier to dive into the stream of love than to get out of it.

Letters passed. Almost all are Madeleine Smith's, for his were no doubt destroyed. They are a revelation of what passion can do. Not to read these letters is not to understand Madeleine Smith.

MY DEAR EMILE,

I do not feel as if I were writing to you for the first time. Though our intercourse has been very short, yet we have become as familiar friends. May we long continue so. And ere long may you be a friend of Papa's is my most earnest desire. We feel it rather dull here after the excitement of a town's life. But then we have much more time to devote to study and improvement. I often wish you were near us, we could take such charming walks. One enjoys walking with a pleasant companion, and where could we find one equal to yourself?

I am trying to break myself of all my *very* bad habits, it is you I have to thank for this, which I do sincerely from my heart. Your flower is fading.

> 'I never cast a flower away,
>   The gift of one who cared for me
> A little flower, a faded flower.
>   But it was done reluctantly.'

I wish I understood Botany for your sake, as I might send you some specimens of moss. But alas! I know nothing of that study. We shall be in Town next week. We are going to the Ball on the 20th of this month, so we will be several times in Glasgow before that. Papa and Mama are not going to town next Sunday. So of course you do *not* come to Row. We shall not expect you. Bessie desires me to remember her to you. Write on Wednesday or Thursday. I must now say adieu.

With kind love, believe me,
Your very sincerely,
MADELEINE.

(Dated 3rd April, 1855).

MY DEAR EMILE,

Many thanks for your kind epistle. We are to be in town to-morrow (Wednesday). Bessie said I was not to let you know. But I must tell you why! Well, some friend was kind enough to tell papa that you were in the habit of walking with us. Papa was very angry with me for walking with a gentleman unknown to him. I told him he had been introduced and I saw no harm in it. Bessie joins with Papa and blames me for the whole affair.

She does not know I am writing you, so don't mention it. We are to call at our old quarters in the Square on Wednesday about quarter past 12 o'c. So if you could be in Mr McCall's lodgings—see us come out of Mrs Ramsay's—come after us—say you are astonished to see us in Town without letting you know—and we shall see how Bessie acts. She says she is not going to write you. We are to be in Town all night. We are to be with Mrs Anderson. Rest assured I shall not mention to anyone that you have written me. I know from experience that the world is not lenient in its observations. But I don't care for the world's remarks so long as my own heart tells me I am doing nothing wrong. Only if the day is fine expect us to-morrow. Not a word of this letter. Adieu till we meet. Believe me, yours most sincerely.
      MADELEINE.

MY DEAR EMILE,
    I now perform the promise I made in parting to write you soon. We are to be in Glasgow to-morrow (Thursday). But as my time shall not be at my own disposal I cannot fix any time to see you. Chance may throw you in my way.
    I think you will agree with me in what I intend proposing, viz.: That for the present the correspondence had better *stop*. I know your good feeling will not take this unkind, it is meant quite the reverse. By continuing to correspond harm may arise. In *dis*continuing it nothing can be said. It would have afforded me great pleasure to have placed your name on. . . .

That letter was not read further in the court.

L'Angelier was not to be cast aside with ease. He replied:

'In the first place I did not deserve to be treated as you have done. How you astonish me by writing such a note without condescending to explain the reasons why your father refuses to consent. He must have reasons, and I am not allowed to clear myself of accusations.

I should have written you before, but I preferred waiting until I got over surprise your last letter caused me, and also to be able to write to you in a calm and collected manner, free from any animosity whatever.

Never, dear Madeleine, could I have believed you were capable of such conduct. I thought and believe you unfit for such a step. I believed you true to your *honour*. I will put questions to you, which answer to yourself. What would you think if even one of your servants had played with anyone's affections as you have done, or what would you say to hear that any lady friends had done what you have—or what am I to think of you now. What is your opinion of your own self after those solemn vows you uttered and wrote to me. Show my letters to anyone, Madeleine, I don't care who, and if any find that I misled you I will free you from all blame. I warned you repeatedly not to be rash in your engagement and vows to me, but you persisted in that false and deceitful flirtation, playing with affections which you knew to be pure and undivided, and knowing at the same time that at a word from your father you would break all your engagement.

You have deceived your father as you have deceived me. You never told him how solemnly you bound yourself to me, or if you had, for the honour of his daughter he could not have asked to break off an engagement as ours. Madeleine, you have truly acted wrong. May this be a lesson to you never to trifle with any again. I wish you every happiness. I shall be truly happy to hear that you are happy with another. You desire and now you are at liberty to recognize or cut me just as you wish—but I give you my word of honour I shall act always as a gentleman towards you. We may meet yet, as my intentions of going to Lima are now at an end. I would have gone for your sake. Yes, I would have sacrificed all to have you with me, and to leave Glasgow and your friends you detested so very much. Think what your father would say if I lent him your letters for a perusal. Do you think he would sanction your breaking your promises. No, Madeleine, I leave your conscience to speak for itself.

I flatter myself he can only accuse me of a want of fortune. But he must remember he too had to begin the world with dark clouds round him.

I cannot put it into my mind that you are yet at the bottom of all this.'

A letter to him from her seems to have ignored this estrangement. It may have been wrongly numbered. The next one suggests the complete break.

DEAREST MISS PERRY,

Many kind thanks for all your kindness to me. Emile will tell you I have bid him adieu. My papa would not give his consent so I am in duty bound to obey him, comfort dear Emile. It is a heavy blow to us both. I had hoped some day to have been happy with him, but alas it was not intended. We were doomed to be disappointed. You have been a kind friend to him. Oh! Continue so. I hope and trust he may prosper in the step he is about to take. I am glad now that he is leaving this country, for it would have caused me great pain to have to meet him. Think my conduct not unkind. I have a father to please and a kind father too. Farewell, dear Miss Perry, and with much love,

  Believe me,
   Yours most sincerely,
   MIMI.

Most of these letters were undated, but the first was written on the 3rd of April, 1855. It showed the bud of friendship. The one we have just quoted suggests that in the bud was a canker. But the next, bearing the post-mark September 4th, 1855, has a dramatic turn that can scarcely have been expected after the epistle to Miss Perry.

MY DEAREST EMILE,

How I long to see you. It looks an age since I bid you adieu. Will you be able to come down the Sunday after next? You will be in Town by 14th. I do not intend to say anything till I have seen you. I shall be guided by your entirely, and who could be a better guide to me than my intended husband. I hope you have given up all idea of going to Lima. I will never be allowed to go to Lima with you—so I shall fancy you want to get quit of your Mimi. You can get plenty of appointments in Europe—any place in Europe. For my sake do not go. . . . I am quite tired of company. What would I not give for to be with you alone. Oh! Would we not be happy. Ah! Happy as the day was long. Give dear Miss P. my love and a kiss when you write. I love her so. What a friend she would be to us. I feel well since I got your last letter, and I try to appear cheerful before my family, and it is not easy to appear in good spirits when there is a pain at the heart. It will break my heart if you go away. You know not how I love you, Emile. I live for you alone. I adore you. I never could love another as I do you. Oh! dearest Emile, would I might clasp you now to my heart. Adieu for to-day—if I have time I shall write another note—before I post this. If not—I shall have a letter at the Garden for you. So adieu, dearest love, and a fond embrace.

Believe me your ever devoted and fond
MIMI.

The next day she wrote again and sent 'a kiss', the first she has given him by letter.

After the temporary set-back, when she attempted to break off the understanding or engagement, she has returned with heated heart to the connection. The following letter was written on December 3rd:

My own darling husband,

I am afraid I may be too late to write you this evening, so as all are out I shall do it now my sweet one. I did not expect the pleasure of seeing you last evening, of being *fondeled* by you, dear, dear Emile. Our cook was ill and went to bed at 10—that was the reason I could see you—but I trust ere long to have a long long interview with you sweet one of my soul, my love, my all, my own best beloved. I hope you slept well last evening and find yourself better to-day. . . . Never fear me. I love you well, my own sweet darling Emile. Do go to Edr. and visit the Lanes—also, my sweet love, go to the ball given to the officers. I think you should consult Dr McFarlan—that is, go and see him; get him to sound you—tell you what is wrong with you. Ask him to prescribe for you—and, if you have any love for your Mimi, follow his advice and oh! Sweet love, do not try and Dr yourself—but oh, sweet love, follow the M.D. advice be good for once and I am sure you will be well. . . . This is a horrid scroll as I have been stopped twice with that bore, visitors. My own sweet beloved, I can say nothing as to our marriage as it is not certain when they may go from home, or when I may go to Edr. it is uncertain. My beloved, will we require to be married (if it is in Edr.) in Edr. or will it do here? You know I

know nothing of these things. I fear the banns in Glasgow there are so many people know me. If I had any other name but Madeleine it might pass—but it is not a very common one. But we must manage in some way to be united ere we leave Town. . . . I shall never forget the first visit I payed with my own beloved husband, my own sweet dear Emile—you sweet dear darling. If ever I again show temper (which I hope to God I won't) don't mind it—it is not with you I am cross. Sweet love, I adore you with my heart and soul. I must have a letter from you soon. I am engaged up till Friday night. Sweet pet, will that be too soon for you to write. . . . When may be may we meet again—soon soon I hope and trust. Sweet darling, you are kind to me, very kind and loving. I ought never in any way to vex or annoy you. . . . Much much love, kisses, tender long embraces, kisses, love. I am thy own, thy ever fond, thy own dear loving wife, thy
MIMI L'ANGELIER.

That's the clarion note of love. These people were writing and meeting clandestinely. One can almost see her with eager eyes, waiting for the next encounter. There is the hint of the physical in the *fondeled*, the kisses, the embraces. After all, love is physical.

Through the winter this secret engagement was carried on, with no diminution in her fervour. It would have been interesting to read his letters, but they were destroyed.

This tell-tale epistle was written about the 7th of May, 1856, at 5 o'clock in the morning:

My OWN, MY BELOVED HUSBAND,

I trust to God you got home safe and were not much the worse of being out. Thank you my love for coming so far to see your Mimi. It is truly a pleasure to see you, my Emile. Beloved if we did wrong last night it was in the excitement of our love. Yes beloved I did truly love you with my soul. I was happy, it was a pleasure to be with you. Oh! if we could have remained never more to be parted. But we must hope the time shall come. I must have been very stupid to you last night. But everything goes out of my head when I see you my darling, my love. I often think I must be very very stupid in your eyes. You must be disappointed with me. I wonder you like me in the least. But I trust and pray the day may come when you shall like me better. Beloved, we shall wait till you are quite ready. I shall see and speak to Jack on Sunday. I shall consider about telling Mama. But I don't see any hope from her—I know her mind. You, of course, cannot judge of my parents. You know them not. . . . Darling Emile, did I seem cold to you last night? Darling, I love you. Yes, my own Emile I love you with my heart and soul. Am I not your wife? Yes I am. And you may rest assured after what has passed I cannot be the wife of any other but dear dear Emile. No, now it would be a sin. . . . I dread next winter. Only fancy beloved us both in the same town and unable to write or see each other; it breaks my heart to think of it. Why, beloved, are we so unfortunate? I thank you very much for your dear long letter. You were kind to me love. I am sorry for your cold. You were not well last night; I saw you were not yourself. Beloved pet take care of it. When may we meet (Oh! that blot!) again? A long time—is it not sad? I weep to think of it; to be separated thus; fi you were far away it would not be so bad—but to think you near me. . . . Emile, beloved, I have sometimes thought would you not like to go to Lima after we are married? Would that not do? Any place with you pet. I did not bleed in the least last night—but I had a good deal of pain during the night. Tell me pet, were you angry at me for allowing you to do what you did, was it very bad for me? We should, I suppose, have waited till we were married. I shall always remember last night. Will we not often talk of our evening meetings after we are married. Why do you say in your letter—'If we are *not* married?' I would not regret knowing you. Beloved, have you a doubt but that we shall be married some day. I shall write dear Mary soon. What would she say if she knew we were so intimate—lose all her good opinion of us both—would she not? My kind love to your sisters when you write. Tell me the names of your sisters. They shall be my sisters some day. I shall love if they are like their dear brother, my dear husband. I know you can have little confidence in me. But dear, I shall not flirt. I do not think it is right of me. I should only be pleasant to gentlemen. Free with none my pet in conversation but yourself. . . . Adieu again my dear husband. God bless you and make you well. And may you yet be very very happy with your Mimi as your little wife. Kindest fond love embrace and kisses from thy own true and ever devoted Mimi thy faithful

WIFE.

The following was found in L'Angelier's lodgings, and the court decided it could not be read as it was not signed, and there was no evidence of it—or a copy—having been sent by post. As it was clearly written by L'Angelier we will quote it as it helps us to see his view-point.

MY DEAREST AND BELOVED WIFE MIMI,

I got home quite safe after leaving you, but I think it did my cold no good. I was fearfully excited the whole night. I was truly happy with you my pet; too much so, for I am now too sad. I wish from the bottom of my heart we had not been parted. Though we have sinned, ask earnestly God's forgiveness and blessings that all the obstacles in our way may be removed from us. I was disppointed, my love, at the little you had to say but I can understand why. You are not stupid, Mimi, and if you disappoint me in information, and I have cause to reproach you of it, you will have no one to blame but yourself. Sometimes I think you take no notice of my wishes and desires but say yes for mere matter of form. Mimi, unless Huggins helps me I cannot see how I shall be able to marry you for years. What misery to have a future in one's mind. Do speak to your brother, open your heart to him, and try and win his friendship. Tell him if he loves you to take your part. And besides, my dear, if once you can trust how pleasant it would be for you and me to meet. I could come over to Helensburgh when you would be riding or driving or of a sunday. Mimi dearest, you must take a bold step to be my wife. I entreat you pet, by the love you have for me Mimi, do speak to your mother—tell her it is the last time you ever shall speak of me to her. You are right, Mimi, you cannot be the wife of anyone else than me. I shall ever blame myself for what has taken place. I never never can be happy until you are my own, my dear fond wife. Oh! Mimi, be bold for once, do not fear them—tell them you are my wife before God. Do not let them leave you without being married, for I cannot answer what would happen. My conscience reproaches me of a sin that marriage can only efface. . . . We must not be separated all next winter, for I know Mimi, you will be as giddy as last. You will be going to public balls and that I cannot endure. On my honour, dearest, sooner than see you or hear of you running about as you did last, I would leave Glasgow myself. Though I have truly forgiven you. I do not forget the misery I endured for your sake. . . .

The date of the foregoing was probably June. The date of the next was about June 14th.

My own, my darling husband,
    To-morrow night by this time I shall be in possession of your dear letter. I shall kiss it and press it to my bosom. Hearing from you is my greatest pleasure: it is next to seeing you my sweet love. My fond Emile—Are you well, darling of my soul? . . . I am longing to see you my sweet pet—to kiss and pet you. Oh! for the day when I could do so at any time. I fear we shall spoil each other when we are married, we shall be so loving and kind. We shall be so happy happy—in our own little room—no one to annoy us—to disturb us. All to ourselves we shall so enjoy that life. . . .
                                        I'm thy Wife, they own true
                                                    MIMI.

The first P.S. ended: 'A kiss dear love from thy devoted and loving, much attached wife, thine own, Mimi.'

The second P.S. ended: 'I am thine until death do separate us, they Mimi.'

The next bore the postmark of Helensburg, June 27, 1856:

                                                    Friday night
    Beloved, dearly beloved husband, sweet Emile. How I long to call you mine, never more to leave you. What must occur ere that takes place God only knows. I often fear some cloud may yet fall on our path and mar our happiness for a long time. I shall never cause you unhappiness again. No,

I was unkind, cruel, unloving—but it shall never be repeated. No, I am now a wife, a wife in every sense of the word, and it is my duty to conduct myself as such. Yes, I shall behave now more to your mind. . . . Your income would be quite enough for me—don't for a moment fancy I want you to better your income for me—no dearest, I am quite content with the sum you named. When I first loved you I knew you were poor. I felt then I would be content with your lot however humble it might be. Yes. Your home in whatever place, or whatever kind, would suit me. If you only saw me now—I am all alone in my little bedroom—you would never mention your home as being humble. I have a small room on the ground floor, very small—so don't fancy I could not put up in small rooms, and with humble fare. . . . Oh how I love that name of Mimi. You shall always call me by that name—and dearest Emile if ever we should have a daughter I should like you to allow me to call her Mimi for her father's sake. You like that name and I love it. . . .

HELENSBURG postmark.
July 15, 1856.

MY SWEET BELOVED AND DEAREST EMILE,

I shall begin and answer your dear long letter. In the first place, how are you? Better I trust. You know I did feel disappointed at our marriage not taking place in Sp!   Emile, dear husband, how can you express such words—that you mar my amusements—that you are a bore to me. Fie, fie, dear Emile. You must not say so again—you must not even think so, it is so very unkind of you. Why I would be very unhappy if you were not near me. . . . Our intimacy has not been *criminal* as I am your wife before God—SO IT HAS BEEN NO SIN—our loving each other. No, darling fond Emile I am your wife. . . .

Date, July, 1856.

BELOVED AND DARLING HUSBAND DEAR EMILE,

I have just received your letter. A thousand thanks for it. It is kind and I shall love you more for writing me such a letter. Dearest I do love you for telling me all you think of me. Emile I am sorry you are ill. I trust to God you are better. . . . Yes Emile, you ought in those sad moments to consider you have a wife. I am as much your wife as if we had been married a year. You cannot—will not leave—me, your wife. Oh! For pity's sake do not go. I will do all you ask—only remain in this country. I shall keep all my promises. I shall not be thoughtless and indifferent to you. On my soul I love you and adore you with the love of a wife. I will do anything—I will do all you mention in your letter—to please you—only do not leave me or forsake. I entreat of you, my husband, my fondly loved Emile, only stay and be my guide, my husband dear. You are my all—my only dear love. Have confidence in me sweet pet. Trust me. Heaven is my witness I shall never prove untrue to you—I shall—I am your wife. No other one shall I ever marry. . . . I adore you with my heart and soul. Emile, I swear to you I shall do all you wish and ask me. I love you more

than life. I am thine. Thine own Mimi L'Angelier. Emile, you shall *have
all* your letters the first time we meet. It may cost me a sigh and a pang, but
you shall have them all. . . . Minnoch left this morning—say nothing to
him in passing. It will only give him cause to say you did not behave in a
gentlemanly manner. Do not do it. He said nothing to me out of
place—but I was not a moment with him by myself. I did not wish to be
alone with him. . . . Love, my pet, my husband, my fond and ever dearly
beloved Emile. Good-night. May God grant you better health. Be happy.
Adieu, sweet one. I am thy wife, thy own fond pet—
                    MADELEINE SMITH,
                    alias MIMI L'ANGELIER.

                                        Date about *August* 14, 1856.

BELOVED AND EVER DEAR EMILE,
    All by myself. So I shall write to you dear husband. Your visit of last
night is over. I longed for it. How fast it passed—it looked but a few
minutes ere you left me. You did, love, look cross at first, but thank
Heaven you looked yourself ere you left—your old smile. Dear fond
Emile I love you more and more. Emile, I know you will not go away from
me. I am your wife. You cannot leave me for ever. Could you Emile? I
spoke in jest of your going last night. For I do not think you will go very far
away from me Emile, your wife. Would you leave me to the end of my days
in misery? For I can never be the wife of another, after our intimacy. But,
sweet love, I do not regret that—never did and never shall. Emile, you
were not pleased because I would not let you *love* me last night. Your last
visit you said, 'You would not do it again till we were married. . . .' No
would not do it again till we were married. . . .' No one heard you last
night. Next night—it shall be a different window—that one is much too
small.

Probably the next letter in sequence, but the post-mark was obliter-
ated. This is interesting because it lets us see what she read and it
mentions Mr Minnoch:

MY OWN DEAR EMILE,
    Now must I thank you for your kind dear letter. Accept a fond embrace
and dear kisses and assurances that I love you as much as ever and have
never regretted what has occurred. I forgive you freely from my heart for
that picture; never do the same thing again. . . . I told you what I liked in
the August *Blackwood*. I shall read the Sept. one on Monday. I think you
should not mind getting a Ring but you shall have the size. I don't know
which finger it ought to be I am sure. I have never noticed these things. I
did tell you at one time that I did not like William Minnoch, but he was so
pleasant that he quite raised himself in my estimation. I wrote to his
sisters to see if they would come and visit us next week, also him, but they

cannot. . . . You ask me what I have been reading. Well then I shall tell you. The lives of 'Leonardo de Vinci' and 'M. Angelo' and 'Andrea del Sarto'—all first-class painters. I am fond of reading the lives of painters. The life of Andrea del Sarto quite makes me feel melancholy. His life was a life of unhappiness—he was a prey to sorrow—he never knew what it was to be happy. . . .'

From a letter dated about October 8th, 1856:

'. . . I know you will, I feel sure you will quarrel with me this winter. I know it well, sweet love—but only know dearest, that I have no desire ever to be parted from you, so Emile, my own sweet Emile, if we should ever part it will be on your side, not mine. I sometimes fancy you are disappointed with me. I am not what you once thought I was. I am too much of a child to please you. I am too fond of amusement to suit your fancy. I am too indifferent, and I do not mind what the world says, not in the least—I never did. I promise to marry you knowing I would never have my father's consent. I would be obliged to marry you in a clandestine way; I knew you were poor. All these I do not mind. I knew the world would condemn me for it, but I did not mind. I trust you have days of happiness before us—but God knows we have days of misery too. Emile, my own, my ever dear husband, I have suffered much on your account from my family. They have laughed at my love for you—they taunted me regarding you. I was watched all last winter. I was not allowed out by myself for fear I should meet you—but if I can I shall cheat them this winter.'

And so these letters go on. Her passion and rapture are not abated. Towards the end of January, 1857, she wrote:

Sunday night, ½ past 11 o'c.

EMILE, MY OWN BELOVED,

You have just left me. Oh, sweet darling, at this moment my heart and soul burns with love for thee; my husband, my own sweet one. Emile, what would I not give at this moment to be your fond wife? We would be happy. Emile, I adore you. I love you with my heart and soul. I do vex and annoy you, but oh! sweet love, I do fondly truly love you with my soul to be your wife, your own sweet wife. . . .'

And the next letter was this. Suggested date, early February, *1857.*

I felt truly astonished to have my last letter returned to me. But it will be the last you shall have an opportunity of returning to me. When you are not pleased with the letters I send you, then our correspondence shall be at an end, and as there is coolness on both sides our engagement had better be broken. This may astonish you, but you have more than once returned me my letters, and my mind was made up that I should not stand the same thing again. And you also annoyed me much on Saturday by your conduct in coming so near me. Altogether I think owing to coolness and indifference (nothing else) that we had better for the future consider ourselves as strangers. I trust to your honour as a gentleman that you will not reveal any thing that may have passed between us. I shall feel obliged by your bringing me my letters and likeness on Thursday evening at 7—be at the Area Gate and C.H. will take the parcel from you. I trust you may yet be happy and get one more worthy of you than I. On Thursday at 7 o'c.

I am, etc.,

M.

You may be astonished at this sudden change—but for some time back you must have noticed a coolness in my notes. My love for you has ceased and that is why I was cool. I did once love you truly, fondly, but for some time back I have lost much of that love. There is no other reason for my conduct, and I think it but fair to let you know this. I might have gone on and become your wife, but I could not have loved you as I ought. My conduct you will condemn, but I did at one time love you with heart and soul. It has cost me much to tell you this—sleepless nights, but it is necessary you should know. If you remain in Glasgow or go away, I hope you may succeed in all your endeavours. I know you will never injure the character of one you so fondly love. No, Emile I know you have honour and are a Gentleman. What has passed you will not mention. I know when I ask you that you will comply. Adieu.'

'Astonished at this sudden charge! ' One would certainly guess that. Not more than a fortnight before she was his 'own dear, sweet little pet wife', and now 'I am, etc. M.'

Astonished! He was more than astonished.

It is worth while trying to understand what has really happened.

Madeleine Smith, the daughter of a well-to-do Glasgow architect, was clearly a romantic creature very much in love with love. The romantic note is struck now and then in her phrases 'You know them not.' 'Ere this. . . .' Her eyes are gazing for romance. But she had much more in her than a thirst for romance.

And this man, L'Angelier, was a woman chaser. It is ours merely to set down what we believe to be true. Mr E.V. Mackay, a Dublin merchant, said he had seen quite enough of L'Angelier to enable him to form an opinion of his character and disposition: 'I formed anything but a good opinion of him. I considered him a vain, lying fellow. He was very boastful of his personal appearance and parties admiring him, ladies particularly. . . . He said ladies admired him very often. I remember one occasion particularly, when he came in when I was reading the papers in the Rainbow. He told me he had met a lady in Princes Street with another lady, and she had remarked to her companion what pretty little feet he had. I had said he was a rather pretty little person, and he had gone out and concoted the story of the lady's remark. I never believed anything he said afterwards.'

Someone else thought him 'rather a forward man and full of pretension.' And someone else, 'well-behaved, well-principled, religious.'

Industrious, ambitious, probably agreeable in conversation, vain, religious and somewhat carnal—that may sum him up.

And it was this man L'Angelier, who thrust himself, with true Gallic audacity in love matters, on to Madeleine Smith, when she was in a mood to regard a man as a prince in disguise.

The letters have told us what happened. But the 'how' is interesting. Letters were addressed to a Miss Perry, a friend of L'Angelier. The lovers met—and met at the Smiths' house! Her daring was amazing and is an indication of her character. She actually let this man L'Angelier into the house—probably into her room, certainly into the laundry and the drawing-room—when her parents had no idea that she was having anything at all to do with him. She was helped by one of the servants, 'C.H.'—Christina Haggart. But she didn't need help. This is from her letter of the 21st November.

'If Mama and Papa were from home I would take you in very well at the front door, just the same way as I did in India Street, and I won't let a chance pass . . .'

So we get the story of the letters and visits. The Smiths were not always in Glasgow, but L'Angelier was willing to travel any distance to see his Mimi.

That he should regard the capture of the daughter of a rich Glasgow architect with pride was natural. The opposition of the parents was something to be got over. His small salary was also more than a reproach. He would probably have been glad of a runaway match with the hope of the parents recognizing the inevitable, for he certainly fixed a date for the wedding.

And then this jilting blow came. What had happened?

Madeleine Smith had become engaged to a Mr William Minnoch— the name appears in sundry letters—on January 28th, 1857. Mr Minnoch had been paying his addresses to her for some time. Mr Smith probably favoured the match. Mr Minnoch was a well-to-do merchant, older than Madeleine Smith, but suggesting romance with all domestic comforts, whereas poor Emile L'Angelier promised a hectic business in a cold room.

No man likes to be jilted. L'Angelier was really in love with Miss Smith; he and she had held each other in the abandon of love and now she writes, 'My love for you has ceased.'

Love doesn't run down quite like a musical-box.

In any case L'Angelier won't take this lying down. What he wrote we don't know because his letters were destroyed, but the appeals on her part came from the heart, even if it was a heart that recked of nothing but self.

EMILE,
I have just had your note. Emile for the love you once had for me do nothing till I see you—for God's sake do not bring your once loved Mimi to an open shame. Emile, I have deceived you. I have deceived my mother . . . I deceived you by telling you she still knew of our engagement. She did not. . . . Emile write to no one, to Papa or any other. Oh! do not till I see you on Wednesday night—be at the Hamiltons at 12, and I shall open my shutter and then you come to the Area Gate, I shall see you. It would break my mother's heart. Oh, Emile be not harsh to me. I am the most guilty, miserable wretch on the fact of the earth. Emile, do not drive me to death. When I ceased to love you, believe me, it was not to love another. I am free from all engagement at present. Emile, for God's sake do not send my letters to Papa. It will be an open rupture. I will leave the house. I will die. Emile do nothing till I see you. . . .

And so on. He had evidently threatened to show her letters to her Papa. She goes on with that writhing pleading. She grovels. Then she reverts to the 'Dearest, Sweet Emile' again. It was 'Bring my letters, darling.' 'Let me have my letters, sweet Emile.'

It was early in February she wrote the cold letter to L'Angelier telling him she no longer loved him. On the 28th of January she had accepted Mr William Minnoch as her future husband. Her plan was clear; she meant by pleading, by cajolery, by any means to get her letters from L'Angelier and stop his mouth.

She tried making love again.

But he had heard she was engaged to Mr Minnoch and was jealous. 'And is it true?' he asked her, 'that you are, directly or indirectly, engaged to Mr Minnoch or to anyone else but me?' He wrote that on

March 5th, so she was playing a dangerous game.

On March 12th Madeleine is with Minnoch at Bridge of Allan and they walk together and talk, together and agree to get married on June 18th.

Mr Minnoch, returning to Glasgow, receives this letter from his betrothed from Bridge of Allan:

> MY DEAREST WILLIAM,
>
> It is but fair, after your kindness to me that I should write you a note. The day I part from friends I always feel sad, but to part from one I love, as I do you, makes me feel truly sad and dull. . . . My aim through life shall be to please and study you. . . . Accept my warmest, kindest love, and ever believe me to be yours with affection.
>
> MADELEINE.

On the 19th she dined with her father and mother at Mr Minnoch's and went with him to the opera. She got home about 11 o'clock. And she had fixed a meeting with L'Angelier at midnight to whom she was writing about that time as 'Dearest and Beloved . . . Sweet one of my heart, my only dear love . . . Ever yours with love and fond kisses . . .'

Some dates are useful.

On January 28th Madeleine Smith became engaged to William Minnoch.

Early in February she decided to break off with L'Angelier.

And also early in February—between the 6th and the 12th—she sent a boy, who acted as page in the family, to buy a bottle of prussic acid.

A firm of druggists had this entry on February 21st.

'Miss Smith, 7 Blythswood Square, 6d. worth of arsenic for garden and country house. M.H. Smith.'

L'Angelier was the jealous man. Minnoch was the happy man. Madeleine Smith was the tortured soul, for she wanted to marry Minnoch and had called L'Angelier her husband. No wonder the letters between Madeleine Smith and L'Angelier are scorching.

He had already spoken of the whole matter to a Mr Kennedy, the cashier at Huggins & Co. He told him that he had been asked to return her letters and said he would never allow her to marry another man as long as he lived. 'She will be the death of me,' he said.

In February he was ill and vomited. He told his landlady he had been taken ill on the road home. She fixed the date of the second illness about

February 22nd and the first one about a week before. He got leave from business and went to Edinburgh. When he returned to Glasgow on the 17th of March he was naturally eager to get a letter. There was none.

So on Thursday the 19th he went to Bridge of Allan. And when he had gone the letter came. It was forwarded to him and he was back in Glasgow on Sunday, much to the surprise of his landlady. 'The letter brought me home,' he said in answer to her question. He had walked fifteen miles then. He was looking well. And, after all, a fifteen mile walk was a fair test of his health. He went out that night at nine o'clock and suggested he might be late.

What had taken him out?

We have not all the evidence, but the missed interview, probably due to the missed letter, is explained by this letter which was posted in Glasgow on the 21st of March and delivered the same afternoon.

'Why my beloved did you not come to me. Oh, beloved are you ill? Come to me, sweet one. I waited and waited for you, but you came not. I shall wait again to-morrow night same hour and arrangement. Do come sweet love, my own dear love of a sweetheart. Come beloved and clasp me to your heart. Come and we shall be happy. A kiss fond love. Adieu with tender embraces ever believe me to be your own

Ever dear fond,
MIMI.

And she has already asked Miss Buchanan to be her bridesmaid when she marries William Minnoch in June.

L'Angelier went to that interview. He never told what happened. Mrs Ann Jenkins's story lets us see the end of Emile L'Angelier.

'He took tea and toast that Sunday night,' she said. 'I cannot say what he had on when he went out on Sunday nor when he came in next morning. The gas was out in the lobby, and when I went into the bedroom he was half undressed. He said he had been very bad but he did not say what it was; nor did he say he had been vomiting on the way home. After he came back he vomited a great quantity of stuff. The chamber pot was quite full, but he did not vomit much after I emptied it. He purged twice, once before I went for the doctor and once after. I gave him hot water, he vomited much, and got better. That was before the chamber-pot was emptied, which was done after the doctor came and by his orders. Before he came I told L'Angelier I would keep what he had vomited and let the doctor see it ... Dr Steven assured me that L'Angelier would get over it the same as before. I think on the morning of his death he complained of his throat, but I cannot say. . . . His right hand was clenched when he died.'

He was between twenty-eight and thirty years of age. Madeleine Smith was then twenty-one.

L'Angelier's friends were communicated with; they took possession of those letters. The last one beginning, 'Why my beloved did you not come to me ...' was found in his pocket. Messrs Huggins & Co., L'Angelier's employers, requested Drs Thomson and Steven to make a post-mortem examination of the body. The stomach being tied at both extremities was removed for chemical analysis. Dr Penny, Professor of Chemistry in the Andersonian University, Glasgow, analyzed the stomach and the liquid that had been contained in it. He made a detailed report and came to these conclusions:

'Having carefully considered the results of this investigation I am clearly of opinion that they are conclusive in showing:
First. That the matters subjected to examination and analysis contained arsenic; and
Secondly. That the quantity of arsenic found was considerably more than sufficient to destroy life.
All this is true on my soul and conscience.
(Signed) FREDERICK PENNY,
Professor of Chemistry.

The body was exhumed and portions were sent to Dr Penny for analysis. His conclusions were:

1. That the body of the deceased Pierre Emile L'Angelier contained arsenic.
2. That the arsenic must have been taken by or administered to him while living.

Dr Robert Christison confirmed the report with an additional analysis.

There were about 82 grains of arsenic in the stomach.

What of Madeleine Smith during this time?

On Thursday the 26th she bolted. Mr Minnoch called to see her, found she was not in the house; went to search for her in the company of her brother and found her on board a steamer going to Rowaleyn. They drove back together. Yet he was ignorant of her acquaintanceship with L'Angelier. He knew nothing of these terrible letters. She promised to explain it all later. And she, casually, on a subsequent occasion, alluded to the report that L'Angelier had been poisoned with arsenic and remarked that she had been in the habit of buying arsenic, as she had learned at Clapton School that it was good for the complexion.

That day she was arrested.

We get a vision of her before the arrest in the evidence given at the trial by M Auguste Jauvert de Mean, Chancellor to the French Consul in Glasgow. He knew L'Angelier and the Smiths. He also knew of the understanding between L'Angelier and Madeleine, so, on the evening of L'Angelier's death, he called on Mr Smith and told him of the letters from his daughter that had been in the dead man's possession. He continued, 'Having heard some rumours meanwhile, one day I am not sure which, I saw Miss Smith in presence of her mother. I apprised her of the death of L'Angelier. She asked me if it was of my own will that I came to tell her; and I told her it was not so, but that I came at the special request of her father. I asked her if she had seen L'Angelier on Sunday night; she told me she did not see him. I asked her to put me in a position to contradict the statments which were being made as to her relations with L'Angelier. I asked her if she had seen L'Angelier on Sunday night, and she told me she had not. I said to Miss Smith that the best advice that a friend could give to her in the circumstances was to tell the truth about it. . . . Miss Smith then got up from her chair and told me, 'I swear to you, M Mean, that I have not seen L'Angelier, not on that Sunday only, but not for three weeks',—or 'for six weeks', I am not sure which.'

In these glimpses that we have of Madeleine Smith, after the death of the 'darling, adored, husband' we discern not the suspicion of a tear.

On Tuesday the 30th of June, 1857, began the trial of Madeleine Hamilton Smith for having (1) on two separate occasions in February, 1857, administered arsenic, or other poison, to Pierre Emile L'Angelier, with intent to murder him; and (2) on an occasion in March, 1857, by means of poison, did murder Pierre Emile L'Angelier.

The Judges were Lord Justice-Clerk (Hope) and Lords Ivory and Handyside.

Those who appeared on behalf of the crown were, the Lord Advocate, the Solicitor-General, Mr Donald Mackenzie, Advocate-Depute. Crown Agent, Mr J.C. Brodie, W.S. For the defence there were the Dean of Faculty, Mr George Young and Mr Alexr. Moncrieff, advocates.

It was a 'sensational' case. The newspapers had not then captured the big caption habit, but the people were the same. They packed the courthouse and crowded the approaches. There was a tense silence just before the chief figure entered. 'She appeared about half past ten o'clock,' says a contemporary record, 'accompanied by two policemen and a female attendant, and took her seat with the most perfect self-possession. She is probably about twenty years of age, ladylike in appearance, of middle height and fair complexion, and wore a brown silk dress and straw bonnet trimmed with white ribbon. Her features wore an expression indicative of extraordinary nerve; and it was only by those nearest to the dock that any difference could be seen in the manner of the prisoner from that of the surrounding spectators. Throughout the entire proceedings the prisoner manifested the same composure, paying nevertheless the closest attention to every item of the evidence.'

Another description said, 'In the midst of all this excitement, passing through the eager crowd from and to prison, seated at the bar with hundreds of eyes fixed steadily upon her, Madeleine Smith is the only unmoved, cool personage to be seen. From the first moment to the last she has preserved that undaunted, defiant attitude of perfect repose, which has struck every spectator with astonishment. She passed from the cab to the Court-room—or, rather, to the cell beneath the dock— with the air of a belle entering a ball-room. She ascends the narrow staircase leading into the dock with a cool jaunty air, an unveiled countenance, the same perpetual smile—or smirk, rather, for it lacks all the elements of a genuine smile—the same healthy glow of colour and the same confident ease. . . . Miss Smith never ceased surveying all that goes on around her, returning every stare with compound interest, glancing every second minute at the down-turned eyes in the side galleries, and even turning right round upon the reporters immediately behind her to see how they get along with the note-taking, which is carrying her name and deeds into every British home. . . . The Dean of Faculty, her leading counsel, bids her good morning, or says a word to her when the proceedings close for the day, and she smiles so cheerily that you listen to hear her laugh. Whoever speaks, counsel or witness, must be sensible of the fixed, penetrating glance of her large black eye . . .'

Emile L'Angelier had died of poison. Had that poison been given to him by Madeleine Smith?

The prosecution found their difficulty in proving that Madeleine Smith and the deceased had met immediately preceding his attacks.

The indictment charged the prisoner with having administered arsenic to L'Angelier in February as well as in March. It will be remembered that Mrs Jenkins swore to his illness in February.

In L'Angelier's diary, which was not admitted as evidence and therefore was not a matter for the consideration of the jury, there occur these items for February:

Thurs. 19. —Saw Mimi a few minutes. Was very ill during the night.
Fri. 20. —Passed two pleasant hours with M. in the drawing-room.
Sat. 21. —Don't feel well. Went to T.F. Kennedy's.
Sun. 22. —Saw Mimi in drawing-room. Promised me French Bible.
Taken very ill.

Landladies can't remember whether lodgers are out for a couple of hours or more on certain nights, when they are asked weeks and months afterwards. Besides, L'Angelier's visits to Madeleine were kept as secret as possible.

Miss Buchanan swore she had gone to a druggist's shop with Miss Smith on March 6th, when the latter had bought some arsenic.

Mr Murdock, a druggist, swore he had sold arsenic to Miss Smith on February 21st.

Mr Haliburton, assistant to Mr Currie, chemist, said he had sold Miss Smith arsenic on March 6th. She said it was for rats. Christina Haggart said there were no rats at the house in Blythswood Square.

Did that arsenic go to the rats or to Emile L'Angelier?

The witnesses could get no nearer the core than has been suggested.

Madeleine Smith's declaration was as follows:

'My name is Madeleine Smith. I am a native of Glasgow, twenty-one years of age; and I reside with my father, James Smith, architect, at No. 7, Blythswood Square, Glasgow. For about the last two years I have been acquainted with P. Emile L'Angelier, who was in the employment of W.B. Huggins & Co. in Bothwell Street and who lodged at 11, Franklin Place. He recently paid his addresses to me, and I have met with him on a variety of occasions. I learned about his death on the afternoon of Monday, the 23rd March current, from Mamma, to whom it had been mentioned by a lady named Miss Perry, a friend of M L'Angelier. I had not seen M L'Angelier for about three weeks before his death, and the last time I saw him was on a night about half past ten o'clock. On that occasion he tapped at my bedroom window, which is on the ground floor, and fronts Main Street. I talked to him from the window, which is stanchioned outside, and I did not go out to him, nor did he come in to me. This occasion, which as already said, was about three weeks before his death, was the last time I saw him. He was in the habit of writing notes to me, and I was in the habit of replying to him by notes. The last note I wrote to him was on the Friday before his death, viz. Friday, the 20th March current. In consequence of that note I expected him to visit me on Saturday night, the 21st current, at my bedroom window, in the same way as formerly mentioned, but he did not come and sent no notice. There was no tapping at my windows on said Saturday night, or on the following night, being Sunday. . . . I remember giving him some cocoa from my window one night some time ago, but I cannot specify the time particularly. He took the cup in his hand, and barely tasted the contents; and I gave him no bread to it. I was taking some cocoa myself at the time, and had prepared it myself. . . . As I had attributed his sickness to want of food, I proposed, as stated in the note, to give him a loaf of bread, but I said that merely in a joke and, in point of fact, I never gave him any bread. I have bought arsenic on several occasions. . . . I used it as a cosmetic, and applied it to my face, neck and arms, diluted with water . . . I never administered or caused to be administered to M L'Angelier arsenic or anything injurious. And this I declare to be the truth.

'(Signed) MADELEINE SMITH.'

Counsel did their best. It is agreed that both the prosecution and the defence were at their heights. The Dean of Faculty could let himself go with more fervour than the prosecuting Lord Advocate and he made the utmost of his brief.

This is from the Lord Advocate's address:

'There was an appointment for Thursday the 19th. On Wednesday, the 18th, she bought her third packet of arsenic. She went back to Currie's shop on the 18th, told him that the first rats had been killed, that they had found a great many large ones lying in the house; and, as she had got arsenic before, appeared to be a respectable person, and told her story without hesitation, on the 18th March she got her third packet of arsenic. That letter was enclosed to Thuau to L'Angelier on the same day with the rest. He enclosed it in a letter of his own, in which he says that the letter came at half past twelve, and that he 'hastens to put it into the post if there is time.' L'Angelier got that letter after nine o'clock at Stirling on Sunday morning. He started with a man called Ross in perfect health to walk to Glasgow. He arrived at his lodgings at eight o'clock, and his landlady said he was immensely improved in health. He said a letter had brought him back and his landlady never doubted he was going to visit the lady. He is seen sauntering along in the direction of Blythswood Square about twenty minutes past nine. It is too early. He knows the way of the house and that they have prayers on Sunday night. He must beguile the time a little, and so he goes past Blythswood Square, down to the other side, and makes a call on his acquaintance McAlester, in Terrace Street, but he does not find him at home. The maid-servant recognized him, and says he was there about half past nine. Here my clue fails me; we lose sight of him for the period of two or three hours, and my learned friends on the other side are equally unsuccessful in their endeavours to trace him; but there is no attempt to show that any mortal man saw him anywhere else than the only place he was going to. He went out with the determination of seeing her; and believing that he had an appointment at that place. You cannot doubt that, after coming from the Bridge of Allan, post haste, to see her, walking first from Bridge of Allan to Stirling, then travelling from Stirling to Coatbridge, walking from Coatbridge to Glasgow, and then walking from his lodgings in the direction of Blythswood Square—you cannot believe that he would give up his purpose within a hundred yards of the house. The thing is incredible, impossible. . . . When and how do we see him next? He is found at his own door, without strength to open the latch, at two o'clock in the morning, doubled up with agony, speechless with exhaustion and pain, parched with thirst, and burning with fever; vomiting commences instantly, and the former symptoms, with great aggravations, go on from two till about eleven o'clock when the man dies of arsenic.'

The Dean of Faculty laid emphasis on the fact that L'Angelier's landlady has said he was ill eight or ten days before the 22nd of February. 'You have it proved very distinctly, I think—to an absolute certainty almost—that on the 19th February the prisoner was not in possession of arsenic. . . .' He contended there was no evidence that L'Angelier and the prisoner had met on Sunday evening and that there was much more to be said for suicide than for the prisoner's guilt.

(It may as well be mentioned that L'Angelier was not known to have purchased arsenic.)

The Dean of Faculty read one of Madeleine Smith's passionately pleading letters, while she was engaged to Minnoch and was afraid L'Angelier would go to her father, and then he said, 'Is that the state of mind of a murderess, or can anyone affect that frame of mind? Will you for one minute listen to the suggestion that the letter covers a piece of deceit? No: the finest actress that ever lived could not have written that letter unless she had felt it. And is that the condition in which a woman goes about to compass the death of him whom she has loved? ... A motive to commit a crime must be something a great deal more than the mere fact that the result of that crime might be advantageous to the person committing it. You must see the motive in action and you must see it influencing the conduct before you can deal with it as a motive.'

But we know very well that the 'mere fact that the result of a crime might be advantageous to the person committing it' has been ample motive for many crimes. And in many instances even the bare advantage has been kept naked.

The Dean of Faculty continued: 'On the 28th of January Mr Minnoch proposes, and, if I understand the theory of my learned friend's case aright, from that day the whole character of this girl's mind and feelings was changed, and she set herself to prepare for the perpetration of what my learned friend has called one of the most foul, cool, deliberate murders that ever was committed. Gentlemen, I will not say that such a thing is absolutely impossible, but I shall venture to say it is well nigh incredible. He will be a bold man who will seek to set limits to the depths of human depravity; but this at least all past experience teaches us, that perfection, even in depravity, is not rapidly attained, and that it is not by such short and easy stages as the prosecutor has been able to trace in the career of Madeleine Smith, that a gentle loving girl passed at once into the savage grandeur of a Medea or the appalling wickedness of a Borgia. No, gentlemen, such a thing is not possible. There is and must be a certain progress in guilt, and it is quite out of all human experience, judging from the tone of the letters which I have last read to you, that there should be a sudden transition from affection to the savage desire of removing by any means the obstruction to her wishes and purposes, that the persecutor imputes to the prisoner.'

That may have had its effect on the jury. They had to decide whether a bonny Scotch lassie, belonging to one of the most respectable of families in Glasgow had or had not poisoned a licentious Frenchman. Did she say as she handed him a cup of cocoa, 'Drink this', as she had done before? And was there arsenic in it? Or did they not meet?

The jury found, by a majority, she was not guilty of the first charge in the indictment—that was administering arsenic to L'Angelier in

February. And their verdict on the murder charge was 'Not proven'. Enthusiastic cheering echoed the verdict.

A line of comment on the case from the *Examiner* may be quoted: '. . . But strange and unnatural to say, to Madeleine Smith alone his horrible death seems to have been no shock, no grief, and she demeaned herself on her trial as if L'Angelier had never had a place in her affections. If it had been a trial for poisoning a dog the indifference could not have been greater. . . . After what had passed between her and the deceased L'Angelier, her composure, in our view, wears the aspect of heartless callousness.'

She wrote to a friend, 'I did not feel in the least put about when the jury were out considering whether they should send me home or keep me. I think I must have had several hundred letters, all from Gentlemen, some offering me consolation, and some their hearts and homes. . . .'

She was subsequently married, but not to Mr Minnoch.

Madeleine Smith was lucky.

EDMUND L. PEARSON

Doctor Cream

On a night on October, 1891, a man standing near a public house, in Waterloo Road, London, had his attention attracted by the actions of a girl on the other side of the street. She had been leaning against a wall; suddenly she fell to the ground, flat on her face. In that neighbourhood this was not especially strange, but her observer was a kind-hearted person. He ran across the street, helped her up, and having inquired her address, assisted her to walk home. She was in great distress, but able to say that 'a tall gentleman,' whom she further described, had given her to drink twice 'out of a bottle with white stuff in it.' She was only nineteen; her name, Ellen Donworth; and she belonged to that great army of women who have been pathetically described by almost every English man of letters since De Quincey.

She soon began to suffer frightful convulsions, and although a doctor ordered her removal to a hospital, she died on the way thither. A post-mortem proved poisoning by strychnine. The tragedy caused a great sensation in the neighbourhood, and was called the 'Lambeth mystery.' Nothing more came to light, however, except the receipt of two peculiar letters. One of these, addressed to the coroner, and signed 'A. O'Brien, detective,' offered to reveal the murderer in return for the trifling consideration of £300,000! The other, sent to W.H. Smith & Son in the Strand, accused one of the firm of the crime but offered to save him if the writer, 'H. Bayne,' should be retained as a barrister. The Messrs Smith were further advised to paste a paper in their office window as a sign of acceptance. By request of the police, they put up the paper, but Mr Bayne was coy.

Exactly one week after the murder of Ellen Donworth, people in a house on Lambeth Road were wakened at three in the morning by the screams of a woman. They went to her room, and found her lying across the bed, evidently in great agony. She was a prostitute, a woman of twenty-seven, named Matilda Clover. Earlier in the night she had received in her room a man whom she called 'Fred.' A servant in the house, named Lucy Rose, had seen him arrive, but in the dimly lighted hall got only a glimpse of his tall figure, covered with a cape overcoat, and wearing a high silk hat. Later, she had heard him depart. Clover's torments were appalling, but in an interval of relief she told Lucy Rose that she had been poisoned by some pills given to her by 'that man Fred.' She died, after hours of terrible suffering, and the doctor, by some carelessness, certified that the cause of death was alcoholism.

Late the next month, the distinguished physician, Doctor Broadbent of Portman Square, received an extraordinary letter, signed 'M. Malone.' In it, the doctor was accused of murdering Matilda Clover with strychnine, and threatened with exposure unless he paid over £2,500. He was told, by the writer, to put a 'personal' in the *Daily Chronicle* to signify his willingness to pay the blackmail; and, upon police advice, the advertisement was printed, and the trap laid. 'M. Malone' was invited to call at Doctor Broadbent's house, where two detectives eagerly awaited him. As in the case of the Smiths, however, no attempt was made to follow up the letter. In December, the Countess Russell, at the Savoy Hotel, received a letter in which Lord Russell was accused of the murder of Clover.

After these events, and as in the case of Jack the Ripper, there was an interval of a few months, followed in April by a still greater tragedy. It was enacted, as usual, in a dismal neighbourhood, and in the black hours of night. A police constable walking his beat near the Waterloo Road, at about two in the morning, witnessed the not unusual sight of a man being let out of a house by a young girl. He recognized the latter as one Emma Shrivell, aged about eighteen; and in the light of the street lamp he not only observed that the man was wearing a tall hat, but caught the gleam of eye glasses. Less than an hour later, the house was aroused by shrieks from the Shrivell girl, and from her companion, Alice Marsh. Both were in the tetanic convulsions of strychnine poisoning. They told their landlady that they had been entertaining at supper a man known to them as 'Fred'; he represented himself as a doctor. Before leaving he gave to each girl three 'long, thin pills'—that is, capsules a novelty at that time in England. For some reason the poor creatures obediently swallowed the capsules, and after diabolical tortures descended into the grave. Alice Marsh died in the cab on the way to the hospital; Shrivell endured her sufferings for five hours, and died at eight o'clock.

It was now apparent to the police that they had in London the problem of a systematic murderer; one who operated by poison; and among women to whom any man could have access at any time. An order was issued for the exhumation of the body of Matilda Clover—fourteen coffins had to be moved to reach hers—and an autopsy revealed that she also had died from strychnine. Before long it came to light that many other women had met and talked with the strange man. One of them, called Lou Harvey, afterward wrote a letter to the magistrate describing her curious adventures. She had met the man thrice; the second time was by appointment on the Thames Embankment, where he brought her some pills which he said would improve her complexion. She was suspicious, however, and pretended to take the pills, but actually dropped them on the ground. Meeting her again a month later, he was apparently surprised and disconcerted to find her alive, and quickly walked away.

Another girl upon whom he called used the romantic name of Violet Beverley. To her he offered what he called 'an American drink'—a term which, in the British Isles, has always been practically synonymous with heel-broth. This is not unreasonable when one remembers the perversions of the cocktail which used to be offered at 'American' bars in London and Paris. Miss Beverley was wise and patriotic, and preferred home brews. As a matter of fact, clues to the murderer's detection were becoming numerous—and they were all furnished by the man himself. He was moving about the dark streets of London, grotesque in his high hat and sober professional clothes, but venomous as a puff-adder. It is not unlikely that he formed part of the composite portrait drawn by Mrs Belloc-Lowndes in her extraordinarily able novel, 'The Lodger.' The costume, the Bible-reading, and other peculiarities of the Lodger suggest this idea.

In May, Sergeant McIntyre of Scotland Yard made the acquaintance, by accident, of one Doctor Neill. The officer was introduced to the physician by Mr Armstead, a photographer. Doctor Neill was much annoyed, he said; policemen were following him, suspecting him, and injuring his business. They had even tried to associate him with the deaths of the Marsh and Shrivell girls, when the truth was—said Doctor Neill—that the real culprit was a Doctor Harper. (No official whatsoever had suspected, accused, or followed Doctor Neill.) He had a letter, which had been received by the girls before their deaths, in which they were warned against Doctor Harper, lest he serve them as he had done Matilda Clover and Lou Harvey! This was the first which had been heard of Lou Harvey, and when she was hunted up, she was found alive and well, and able to give some interesting information about Doctor Neill. Other odd events followed, until, early in June, Doctor Neill was arrested for blackmail. Next month, the charge was altered to murder, and in October he came to his trial at the Old Bailey, at the time the District Attorney of Bristol County, Massachusetts, was puzzling himself over the problem of who murdered Mr and Mrs Borden of Fall River.

Thomas Neill Cream, to give the doctor his full baptismal style, may not be the most amazing creature in the history of crimonology, but he was either runner up or in the first group. His career affords some illustration of a saying I once heard (I wish I could trace its source) to the effect that society is at the mercy of a murderer who is remorseless, who takes no accomplices, and who keeps his head. In the last requirement, Neil Cream failed notably: instead, he worked hard to give himself away.

At the time of his arrest he was forty-two years old. Some British writers have described him as 'the American doctor.' There is often a marked tendency, outside this country, to be hazy about the birthplace or political allegiance of such Americans as Sargent, Whistler, and Edwin Abbey—and this is natural. The English journalist, to do him justice, usually awards us Doctor Crippen, but he errs on the side of generosity when he also attributes Doctor Neill Cream to America. A failure of American penal methods did play such a part in the Doctor's adventures, however, that we cannot complain with much vigour.

Cream was born in Glasgow, and his first association with the American continent was when he was four or five. His family, who seem to have been perfectly decent, emigrated to Canada, where, twenty years later, the young man took his degree of doctor of medicine, with merit, at McGill University. He further pursued the study of medicine in London and Edinburgh, where he obtained qualification. Returning to Canada, his actions for the next four or five years were those of a thorough 'wrong 'un.' A marriage contracted at the point of a shotgun in the hands of an indignant parent; frauds on insurance companies; medical and other malpractices with women as their victims; charges of blackmail and of other malodorous deeds, were the principal events of his professional career. He moved to Chicago, but made no change in his scheme of life. His first conviction came in 1881. An elderly man, named Stott, living in Garden Prairie, Illinois, was so foolish as to send to Doctor Cream for his quack remedy for epilepsy. Furthermore, he often sent his pretty young wife to Cream's office in Chicago to make the purchase. Cream's motive in poisoning this man is not clear; it can hardly have been because he wished to legalize his relations with Mrs Stott. As he was trying to insure the life of Stott, it might have been thought—with any rascal less bizarre than Cream—that the object was money. At all events, Mr Stott died twenty minutes after taking one of the doctor's prescriptions, and was buried without suspicion. How great was Mrs Stott's guilty knowledge is a matter of doubt; it is quite possible that she may have been innocent of the murder. Doctor Cream would not let his victim rest in the grave; he insisted, in letters, first to the coroner, and next to the District Attorney, upon an exhumation. This took place, and strychnine was found in the body. Cream was captured, after a flight, and with the woman indicted for murder. She turned State's evidence, and escaped punishment. Cream was found guilty, but in the second degree, and sentenced to imprisonment for life. Illinois in 1881, as in 1924, was carefully saving alive her poisonous serpents.

He was served less than ten years at Joliet. When his father died, in 1887, leaving Doctor Cream some $16,000, sympathizers thought that the time had come to give the poor fellow another chance, with an opportunity to enjoy himself and his inheritance. An agitation was begun to effect his release; Mr Stott was dead, and doubtless anybody who had opposed the commutation would have been denounced as revengeful. The favourite contention of those who wish to let off murderers with an easy punishment, is that a different policy is inspired by vindictiveness. So Governor Joseph W. Fifer of Illinois commuted the sentence; and the Doctor left prison in July, 1891. He visited Canada to gather in his patrimony, and sailed for England, where he landed on October 1st. As with Stevenson's Mr Hyde, his devil had long been caged; he came out roaring. The murder of Ellen Donworth followed on October 13th, and that of Matilda Clover on October 20th.

In the interval following these two murders, and before the others in April, he had made a trip to Canada and the United States. In addition to all the blackmailing letters, and to all the verbal and written threats which he uttered against a number of persons (some of which I have mentioned) he perpetrated, during this trip, one of the strangest of his deeds. He caused to be printed in Quebec 500 copies of a circular, worded as follows:

ELLEN DONWORTH'S DEATH

To the Guests,
of the Metropole Hotel

LADIES AND GENTLEMEN,
I hereby notify you that the person who poisoned Ellen Donworth on the 13th last October is to-day in the employ of the Metropole Hotel and that your lives are in danger as long as you remain in this Hotel.

Yours respectfully,
W.H. MURRAY,

London April 1892

These circulars were sent to him in London, but never used. Nobody has ever discovered their purpose. He brought back with him $1,400 from his father's estate, and celebrated his return with the murder of Marsh and Shrivell.

At his trial, it was impossible to make a strong defence. Girls who saw him with Clover identified him; the constable recognized him as the man whom Shrivell let out of the house. Lou Harvey identified him as the man who had sought to make her take the capsules. He was proved to have written letters in which he said that Clover had died by strychnine, and this at a time when nobody knew the real cause of her death. He was found to be in possession of strychnine; and numerous witnesses, both English and Canadian, told of his frequent conversations about 'operating' among women with that poison. The jury were out only ten minutes before finding him guilty, and on November 15, 1892, the English law carried out the disagreeable task which the law of Illinois had shirked—in the name of humanity—eleven years earlier. That mistaken act of clemency had cost four wretched women torment and death.

What was Neill Cream? By that pseudo-scientific thinking which calls every evildoer insane—on the pretence that we are all naturally good and virtuous—he will, of course, be termed a lunatic. If so, then he was a lunatic for whom the public hangman was the right and proper remedy. The half-horrible and half-absurd novels of the Marquis de Sade are unfamiliar to most modern readers, but since Havelock Ellis wrote 'Studies in the Psychology of Sex' most scientific and many literary folk are familiar with the term sadism; indeed, few novelists of to-day can resist showing their familiarity with it. Nevertheless, Neill Cream, if he delighted in cruelty for its own sake, was of a special and peculiar type: he carefully absented himself from the scene when his victims endured their agonies. He took pains to boast about his crimes, and to advertise them pseudonymously and in ridiculous fashion, as in the Metropole circular. It is asserted that he had been suspected of insanity; he often took drugs—morphine, for instance. In a Court to-day, especially in America, a great fight could be made, on these grounds, to prolong his useless life, and save him for perhaps more deviltry in the future. The tender-hearted preservers of our murderers never give a thought to the future victims of the murderer, nor to the future victims of potential murderers, who note the light penalties which are awarded by mawkishness parading as mercy. The dead are dead, they say; but we must keep these interesting young slayers alive, at Joliet, or elsewhere.

Cream was not insane in a legal sense; he knew the wrong he was doing; he was cool and calm in the transaction of business; none of his London associates through him a lunatic. He would not have murdered had he not believed that he could again outwit the law and escape its penalty. Whatever exactly he was, wrote his biographer, Mr Teignmouth Shore, the halter was his just award.

SIDNEY HORLER
The Hoop-La Murder Trial

This woman may be said to have run the whole gamut of human emotions, not through her own merits but through the stark fact that she was accused of murdering her husband by means of cyanide of potassium poisoning. During her trial she became the most important figure in all the Americas: immediately after the trial she was besieged by film and music-hall agents with dazzling offers—and, final and most bewildering phase of all, two months after her acquittal from an ordeal which a spirited writer in the *New Yorker* called 'as luscious a trial as any in the gaudy annals of American jurisprudence,' she stood beside Mrs Aimée Semple Macpherson, the hot-gospeller revivalist, and sang 'The Old Rugged Cross,' maybe with fervour, but certainly with an eye to the main chance.

If ever a woman can be said to have determined to capitalize the notoriety due to having stood in the dock on a charge of murder, it was Mrs Jessie Costello. She had believed—and hoped—that she would find her inevitable way to the Bright Lights of Broadway as a result of having been placed in the pen; but when the wheel of Fate turned about and landed her instead by the side of that other truly remarkable character, Aimée Semple Macpherson, she felt not only bewildered but reproachful. As the writer in the *New Yorker* so ably put it, 'as she faced 8,000 devout people in Boston's Arena, even the ecstatic amens and hallelujahs that greeted her throaty blues-singer's voice did not completely banish her resentment. Her trial had brought her to God instead of to Broadway, and if she was a bit rebellious who can blame her?'

All things considered, I am of the opinion that the Costello trial—practically unknown in Britain, let it be added—and what followed it constitutes the most amazing piece of criminal jurisprudence within the last fifty years. If any should doubt this assertion, and it is very possible, all I ask is for that sceptic to read on.

The remarkable Jessie was a Maid of Salem. Before her great advancement she strutted on the meagre stage of Peabody, Massachusetts. Peabody is a small, drab, entirely undistinguished factory town of 20,000 inhabitants, distant some thirty miles from Boston. Born in 1902, Jessie had always disliked school, and at the age of fourteen had refused ever to return. She is said to have resembled her father, a breezy, blunt, go-to-hell type of a fellow, with a temper to match his ham-like hands. From an early age—but here I must borrow again the inimitable prose of the *New Yorker* writer:

> Jessie was destined for higher things. The success she achieved at the Salem Court-house was perhaps no surprise to those connoisseurs of seductiveness who, lolling against corner lamp-posts, had watched Mrs Costello's provocative and rather hefty sensuosity wriggle off into the distance. Frequently, in the past, they had given her dark, intense figure, whose ample torso bent a little forward from burgeoning hips, that accolade of approval expressed by the phrase 'get a load of that!' In their way, they were pioneers. Perhaps, too, those of Mrs Costello's neighbours who had engaged with her in certain fierce debates were not surprised by th fire and dash she later revealed. She had a certain masculinity of expression, rich, varied and yet precise, which she occasionally employed in the heat of combat.

From the above, a very good impression will be gathered of the type of woman this was.

She could not settle down to any ordinary employment; perhaps the visions of her future greatness prevented it. In any case, she tripped, in a single year, from a bakery shoppe, to the operation of an adding machine, and from this on to a Peabody Corset Emporium, where she was the chief sales-girl. (With her impressive bust she made a good model, no doubt.)

Well, there Jessie was—an opulent-breasted, big-hipped wench, full of zing, craving for life, never able to stay put for very long in one place, attracting the attention of all the males in the neighbourhood, seeing all the movies, attending all the dances, reading all the highly-spiced sex magazines in which American journalism abounds. It was, we are told, 'a rich, full life'—and it was to be infinitely richer and infinitely fuller.

When she was seventeen—that was in November, 1919—Jessie, looking at least ten years older in spite of the short skirts which were the fashion in those times, attracted the attention, whilst standing on a street corner selling poppies for the disabled veterans of the world war, of a tall, bleak-faced young fireman of Celtic cast, who was walking swiftly by. In the ordinary way, William J. Costello, himself a veteran of the war, and now an employee in the Fire Department of the Peabody Corporation, did not pay any attention to females; he was not that type. Sex meant nothing in his austere life. But this girl was different: when Jessie, reaching out, nabbed him by the arm, passers-by smiled; it was such a characteristic gesture of this go-getting wench. To those who were not beset with arid puritanism, the picture might have been a pleasant one—these onlookers could not have seen the shadow of death hovering in the distance.

Shortly after Jessie pinned a poppy on the coat lapel of William J. Costello, they began courting. Four years later they were married.

Now it does not require a skilled psychologist to opine that a girl of Jessie's characteristics and mentality was a piece of human dynamite to which to be hitched—unless the husband could manage her with a firm hand.

Bill Costello, we are informed, was a bit on the staid side. Compared with his exuberant bride, he looked like one of the Pilgrim Fathers. He had not told the life-loving Jessie beforehand that he spent several hours everyday on his knees; that he was given to brooding not only on his God but on his stomach: for Bill, the fireman, was both religious and suffered from chronic indigestion. Furthermore, Bill was not much of a one for talking. In this he clearly resembled the late President Calvin Coolidge who, when asked by his wife what the Sunday sermon was about, briefly answered: 'Sin,' and when further asked what views the preacher had expounded, coughed up the laconic rejoinder: 'He didn't approve of it.'

To be fair, as every historian should be, I must say that Bill Costello could not have been by any manner of means a lovable character—he was too grim, too rugged, too introspective for that. Apart, altogether, from his unfashionable habit (in these days) of praying for hours on end, his indigestion, and his introspection, he had a somewhat nauseating habit of taking his boots off when he got home from duty and propping his socked feet on the radiator. It does not require much imagination to agree with the *New Yorker* writer already quoted, Mr Richard O. Boyer, that 'Bill had little of the tender sparkle of the heroes Jessie read about in *True Stories*.'

But whatever failings the Peabody fireman possessed, he must have satisfied—at least, for the time being—his wife's requirements as a husband. He did his duty—perhaps grimly, perhaps introspectively, but he did it: after the marriage, we are told, 'there were four children in a sequence almost as swift as biology would allow.'

But children bring diapers—and diapers weren't much in Jessie's line. She regarded them as an unpleasant adjunct of modern civilization. What was more, four young children, all requiring a mother's loving care, cramped her style; she was now no longer the admired girl on the sidewalks; marriage had caught her fast in its toils, and she was buried and lost amidst the multitude of other young housewives of Peabody. It was a melancholy reflection—especially as she had gained forty pounds in weight and had now passed her thirtieth year. Oh, dear!

In a word, Jessie was ripe for mischief when Fate sent across her path the man who was destined to become nationally known as the 'kiss-and-tell-cop.'

This shortly-to-be-blazoned-abroad personage was a pouty-mouthed and tow-haired patrolman (constable, in England) called Edward J. McMahon. This ornament to the Peabody Police Force moved through life in the typically lethargic manner peculiar to his kind; he could aptly, we are told, be described as both mawkish and moon-calfish; nevertheless, he was a great favourite with the ladies. There was, no doubt, a reason.

Almost immediately after our heroine made the acquaintance of McMahon, she was seen to undergo a renaissance. Questioned on the matter, she said—only in plainer, blunter terms—that the relationship between her and the patrolman ('Big Boy') was entirely spiritual, and that she admired McMahon only in a platonic way. When this statement is compared with the astonishing confessions of lecherous intimacy, which McMahon, surely one of the strangest self-accusers who ever stepped into a witness-box, made at the trial, Jessie's love of the truth was, with some degree of fairness, questioned.

But the main thing is that 'Big Boy's' admiration and adoring tactics provided a much-needed tonic for Jessie. She might have posed at this stage of her life, as a 'before' and 'after' witness: if the patrolman had had some rejuvenating pills named after him, his testimony would have sold a wagon-load at every street corner.

Yes, Jessie bloomed again. Once again she came to the forefront, glorying in the limelight. Leaving her dishrags and diapers, she set out to 'go places and do things.' She sold tickets for Policemen's Balls; she participated in Penny Bazaars; she collected funds for the Unemployed, and was a member of several committees. Altogether, a remarkable recrudescence was hers.

'Love had planted roses in her heart,' the newpapers later said. The newspapers *would*. . . .

And then came that fatal February. Up to this time, any thought of a hand of the Law—that same Law with which she was at this time so intimately connected—reaching out to grab her, was unthinkable, but——

The actual date of Jessie's arrest was the 17th of March, 1933. This was exactly a month after the death of her husband, who—poor man!—a long, lank, lugubrious corpse, as in life he had been a long, lank, lugubrious fireman—was found spawled outside the bathroom of his home on Fay Avenue, a rosary lying near it.

In her dim, fumbling way, Jessie had always dreamed of Greatness—and now the newspapers thrust this dubious quality upon her with unstinting hands.

Disregarding the fact that she had passed the age of physical perfection (remember the extra forty pounds motherhood had thrust upon her) it pleased the U.S. journalistic world to portray her as 'Beauty in Distress.' We are informed that 'reporters unable to talk to the widow because of gaol rules, were forced to create their own version of her.' Thus, they thrust upon her all the seductiveness of Helen of Troy, one paper going demented and declaring that 'all the modest sex appeal of Lady Godiva plus clothing but minus horse was hers.' For a few hectic weeks, Jessie thrust all the fashionable film stars away from the front page; she became the shopgirls' ideal. Photographs in abundance were published: 'Male members of lonely hearts' clubs all over the country went to bed thinking of Jessie!'

The Boston Press, usually reflecting the real New England modern puritanism, cast aside all its former restraint and went stark, raving mad. Here was a chance to cash in on their own special sensation and they did so with such wild abandon, that their *confrères* all over the American Continent followed suit. To quote the spirited Mr Boyer once again: 'The Boston Press beat the tom-toms so wildly that their echoes were heard by the journalistic brethren from coast to coast and brought them on the run. Perhaps some genuine *aficionados* of the murder trial ran a bit reluctantly. One might not have expected to find the perfect American trial, with all the hoop-la and idiocies the genre require, in austere New England. Salem, where the House of the Seven Gables still casts its bleak Puritan shadow, seemed to lack the lavishness of temperament that was needed.'

When the alleged murderess (for the charge against Jessie was the specific one of poisoning her husband by means of cyanide of potassium) made her appearance in the dock, she was seen wearing a black dress, ornamented simply with white collar and cuffs. This dress soon became as well known as her smile. (She smiled throughout the trial, let it be added.) The jury, we are told, did not at first display that goggling undisguised admiration that they were to evidence later. They were coy to respond; the Costello magic took time to cast its spell. The bailiff who shortly was to send a bouquet of roses to the prisoner each day, on the opening morning behaved as official decorum dictated; in other words, he looked straight ahead of him and concentrated purely on his duty. Nor did the crowd, who were to cheer Jessie wildly each day as he made her triumphant progress from gaol to court-house, develop these maniacal tendencies until later. In short, the opening morning of the trial gave small indication of the tempest of excitement which was to follow.

Indeed, had it not been for the striking personality of the accused, this might have been just another murder trial. But, and here again I have resource to Mr Boyer,

> facing a possible death sentence, Jessie bloomed like a rose. Her personality dominated the proceedings. Even dull moments seemed to contain a certain breathlessness, a certain lilt, derived, perhaps, from the cadenced hop, skip, jump, wave and smile with which Jessie, four times a day, streaked to and from her limousine through the cheering crowd on her way in and out of the court-house. Then she would pant up the stairway, the fortunates in the building racing in the wake of her broad and straining buttocks. Gaining the second floor, she would stand at the window and wave to the crowd in the street beneath. One day a retinue of vaudeville midgets stood below and received Jessie's wave as if it were a benediction. Their manager henceforth advertised them as The Troupe That Had Been Waved At By Jessie!

Word of the wonderful things that were to be witnessed at the Salem court-house soon got abroad; with his finger characteristically on the American reading-public's pulse, that overlord of the printed word, W.R. Hearst, began to press buttons. He sent such notable United States writers as Will Irwin, Katharine Brush and Adela Rogers St John thither to write their flowing cadences. The Hearst papers, we read, 'were full of typographical aphrodisiacs. Every phrase describing Jessie as a glamorous siren, irresistible to men, seemed to increase the irrelevancy of her guilt or innocence.'

Stimulated by reading such purple prose, was it any wonder that the crowd panting to get into the court-house increased every day—indeed every minute? Once the populace, led by the Press, had firmly come to the opinion that Jessie was the most lovely feminine creature that had been reared in New England for a decade, was it any wonder that the jurors caught the general infection? After all (as Mr Boyer so sapiently points out), they were only men, and Jessie was merely a woman.

Sentiment—mawkish, heavily-scented, sex-pulsating, dreamy-eyed—ruled the camp. Justice went overboard—and who can wonder at it amidst such an atmosphere? It is recorded that one of the jurymen actually inquired if he could send the prisoner a box of candies as a slight gesture of his esteem! So crazy had become the atmosphere of the court-house that, during the recesses, the jurors formed a male voice quartette, and the hot summer air vibrated to their renderings of such songs as 'Sweet Adelaide,' 'My Wild Irish Rose,' and 'Let Me Call You Sweetheart.'

If Jessie became the heroine, her 'Big Boy,' the 'kiss-and-tell-cop,' became the villain—after all, you can't have two heroes in a murder trial: that's asking too much! Even the Hearst papers jibbed at printing all of McMahon's testimony; this was so sizzling in character that strong men were seen to blush, and haughty matrons to (pretend to) swoon. A particularly daring publisher put the moving words into a little red booklet, and this sold in cart-loads. Meanwhile, 'Jessie, heady with adulation and resembling some buxom *prima donna* entering the opera-house amid the cheers of her admirers, cantered through the crowd from limousine to court-house and back again.'

The American male is a chivalrous if simple creature—and seeing Jessie as the heroine of this sordid piece, he commenced to write letters to the prisoner at the rate of five hundred a day. Here are two which were read in Court—both of them in verse, it will be seen.

The first:

> Tear-drops on a velvet rose,
>   Tear-drops—in your eyes,
> Make me wonder if there'll be
>   Tear drops—in Paradise.
> Freedom-home.

ROBERT E. LEE.

The second:

> 'May your life be long and happy,
> May your trouble be but few,
> May you find a home in Heaven,
> When your earthly life is through.'

A Mr J.E. Hazeltine was responsible for this more mature effort.

Mr Hazeltine, whilst pouring out his admiration for Jessie, poured out also a liberal dose of verbal prussic-acid for the man who had confessed that he went to bed with Jessie on innumerable occasions—especially when Bill the foreman was out looking after his fires. He wrote of McMahon in the following blistering words: 'I would not give him a job cleaning out a pig-pen. I would have more respect for the pigs.'

Mr Hazeltine was evidently a deep and profound thinker.

This astoundingly egregious criminal farce wound its way slowly to a close. Every day the radiant happiness of Jessie could be seen depicted more clearly on her dimpled face. For by now there had entered another element: inspired by what they had read in the newspapers, and getting all hot under their vests at the photographs they had seen printed, agents for the burlesque theatre (where 'art' is confined to shapely women provocatively taking off their clothes, piece by piece) arrived on the scene. They all carried contracts in their hands.

Before the Defence had closed its case, there were men in the crowd who talked knowingly of screen tests. Newspapers were said to be prepared to bid fortunes for the rights of Jessie's life story. The Bright Lights of Broadway seemed as inevitable as acquittal when she faced the jury and said simply, but with dignity: 'Gentlemen, send me back to my children.'

How could they—being men with hearts beating—do anything else? Yes, although the most was made of the evidence, Jessie was acquitted.

She came back to the world, her head dizzy with prospective further triumphs: amongst other tangible proofs of her popularity, she had a contract for eleven hundred dollars, representing two appearances daily for four days in a New York theatre. Besides the contract, she had also been provided with a maid, a theatrical agent, two thousand four hundred dollars for the exclusive newspaper rights of her life-story, and two reporters who were to act as her Boswells.

Jessie sped like a meteor—rather a weighty one, with too much flesh round her hips and sagging breasts—towards the Bright Lights of Broadway. In doing so, she disappointed at least one of her admirers—that same Mr Hazeltine, who has been mentioned earlier in this chronicle. Mr Hazeltine was a knight who would not have disgraced himself sitting at King Arthur's table; he had believed that his heroine might struggle for vindication, but never for profit. To commercialize her great ordeal in the way she had done, was something that threatened to break Mr Hazeltine's heart. As for Mr Robert E. Lee, it is said that he talked darkly of taking his life. . . .

America never does anything by halves; this truism was rarely better demonstrated than in the case of Jessie Costello. Contracts were thrust upon Jessie by the handful; they descended upon her like the autumn leaves. And, being so much sought after, Jessie became capricious; amidst the frantic hullabaloo in which she now lived, amidst the never-ceasing, hard, unwinking Bright Lights of Broadway, she turned down scornfully a 20,000 dollar contract for a ten-week burlesque appearance. Her ladylike excuse was that 'she didn't think that taking off her clothes in public was refined,' and so she hurried back to her main occupation—which nowadays was shopping. Feeling that she was a great person in her own right, she conducted it on a lavish scale. 'A dozen pairs of shoes in one place, half a dozen hats in another, silk underwear by the bundle, hosiery, dresses by the score—everything,' was the description one of her reportorial Boswells wrote, swimmy-eyed, in his paper.

Arrayed in all this finery, Jessie did not lead a retired life: on the contrary, she was frequently seen in the fashionable places. In these resorts of the élite she could be seen, 'the cynosure of all eyes, as she sits down in a beautiful gown and ermine wrap, a smart, self-possessed, well-groomed widow.'

When such famous Broadway columnists as Walter Winchell of the New York *Daily Mirror* and Ed Sullivan of the New York *Daily News* came up to be introduced, she was graciousness itself 'as they offered sympathy for the trouble and torture she had been forced to endure.' The picture of Walter Winchell, that hard-boiled commentator on mankind's frailties, offering sympathy for the troubles and tortures which Jessie had endured, should have been photographed—as, no doubt, it was.

Meanwhile Hollywood itself had got busy. Those modern magi, who know what the public wants even before the public has given any indication of it, were gathering in the offing like so many pot-bellied vultures. Presently they descended in shoals, demanding the radiant widow's appearance on the screen.

So here she was, sitting pretty as the saying goes, being besieged by all kinds of *entrepreneurs*. It must have been a gorgeous sight for the observing gods.

Even more gorgeous was the spectacle which almost immediately followed. There was a certain, but as yet inarticulate, portion of the American public, that saw not the trailing clouds of glory, but national disgrace in the acquitted widow's wholesale grabbing of newspaper-space. They resented the fact that a woman who had been accused of murder, and who, according to the man who said he had been her lover, had displayed lascivious tendencies too shocking even to be printed in the newspapers, should be thrust upon the public's consciousness in this manner. They were old-fashioned enough to think that, hidden away somewhere or other, was the merest hint of bad taste. Just a *soupçon*, perhaps, but still there.

So they went to Mr Will Hays, who, as the world knows, was the judge of what shall and shall not be seen in American motion pictures.

Mr Hays, who has been described as 'that great Presbyterian moralist,' saw eye to eye with them. The result was swift, devastating and astonishing; told in plain language that this was one of the things that *must* not be done, the screen magnates lost all interest in the fascinating widow overnight, and the next morning Jessie was left high and dry. All washed up, in fact.

Difficulties now descended upon Mrs Costello, even more quickly than her former successes. It was not to be wondered at, perhaps, that Jessie did not quite understand the difficulties that now lay in her path. She was still artistically obstreperous. She began her second day in the Metropolis, we are told, by

> actually rejecting an 18,000 dollar contract in burlesque, before hurrying out to do some more shopping. She had been about to sign the document, which stipulated 1,600 dollars a week payment for twelve weeks, when her duties were explained—these duties consisted of acting a little scene, 'clean but affectionate' between herself and an actor impersonating the unspeakable McMahon. For an instant Jessie was her old trenchant, eloquent self as she ejected the agent. Then she rushed out and bought a refrigerator, furniture for her six-roomed country cottage, gifts and clothing for her children, and purchases for her friends.

But the thunder-clouds were rapidly gathering; the bad news was broken to Jessie by one of her Boswells that she was no longer saleable. Instantly she changed her front; from being the pursued, she was now the pursuer. No story-book detective could have been more assiduous in tracking down the murderer than she was in tracking down the agents who, warned by Mr Hays, were determined now to have nothing more to do with this bad risk. (As Mr Boyer put it: 'It wasn't fair; it was almost un-American.')

Despairing of the films, she thought twice about the burlesque theatres. Perhaps, after all, what she had been asked to do was not too bad; she went to the manager who had offered her the 18,000 dollar contract referred to above. To her indignant surprise, she was now told that the offer no longer held good. The Bright Lights of Broadway were dimming with a vengeance.

Jessie stood alone.

There was nothing else for it but to return to her Boston home. She returned with no contracts, little money, and a magnificent wardrobe. She returned to find a city of angry critics—and no real friends.

Reaction, you see, had set in; the public had switched their views within an hour. Whereas before there were none so cruel as to impugn her motives, now she found none so brave as to support her. The general comments were summed up in a pregnant phrase by a leader in the campaign for decency. He said:

'Public morals forbid commercializing such a tragic event.'

Determined to snatch what little might remain of her previous astonishing glory, Jessie descended the scale with a sickening thud. No longer able to show herself on stage or dance-hall, she took to the sawdust floor of a Boston public-house. This was owned by Jack Sharkey, the highly temperamental Lithuanian, who had once been heavy-weight champion of the world. In the month of September she entered Sharkey's employ as a 'hostess.'

Then came the most amazing turn-about of this whole epic of hoop-la. Jessie had been working among the sawdust, the spittoons, the drunks and the photographs of other great prize fighters for a fortnight, when she sent word to the local newspapers that she had something to tell them.

The result was this: On October 3rd the local Press carried a statement signed by her to this effect:

I am about to be associated with the noted Los Angeles Evangelist, Mrs Aimée Semple MacPherson.

To quote the fuller details about this staggering prospect, she explained that 'she had gained Sister Aimée's consent and would begin work for the Lord on October 15th, when Sister Aimée would open a revival in Boston.'

In order to dress befittingly for the part, Jessie, we are told, 'bought a becoming nun-like costume of black and went immediately into training.' Her trainer was the Rev Mr William McLam, Boston's Representative of Aimée's nation-wide organization. After a long training session, the Rev Mr McLam emerged into the open and reported progress.

'I'm always glad,' he said to the reporters, 'to co-operative with anyone seeking to enter the Harvest Field. The Master is calling for labourers. We hope Mrs Jessie will come into the great blessing of God's love. I get down on my knees and pray with her.'

Well, what could be fairer than that?

Clemenceau, when he had been a newspaper-man, would have found the opening night of the Revival (Jessie's) a fitting subject for his pen. But even then the withering cynic could not have done justice, perhaps, to this mighty theme.

In the absence of Clemenceau, let us be content with recording the heart-searing words of Mr Boyer:

> When the great night arrived, Sister Aimée's heart must have dropped a beat when she saw her glowing protégée. No one knew better than this aged *prima donna* of the sawdust trail, that the allure which had called so many to God, was beginning to fade. Yet she had retained her coquettish technique. The years that had lined her face had given her such skill that she could sometimes still create the illusion of youth, providing that no younger person stood near.
>
> But now, in the glare of the Boston Arena's lights, she stood before 8,000 people, and, beside the electric Jessie. It was a cruel contrast. The young widow radiated triumph. After many vicissitudes, she had gained an audience. There was something tense, positive, and compelling about her figure. In contrast, Aimée's ageing muscles seemed to sag.

But the old warrior did not go down without a fight.

'I have in mind to-night,' Aimée said, 'a woman who has been separated from her children, and is now finding her way back to God.'

It was unfortunate, no doubt, that her voice sounded thin and reedy; or that her white nurse's uniform, her straw-coloured hair and her pasty face blended with the yellow lights and made her difficult to see: on the other hand, it was even more unfortunate, from her point of view, that Jessie's solid figure was in black.

Aimée continued:

'You must, you know, be broken at the feet of Jesus before you can do anything worth while. Mrs Costello told me, "Oh, sister, I have been broken at the feet of Jesus and think I can help the poor." She told me she'd like to do something for Jesus and that she "didn't want to die empty-handed." '

Called upon to do her stuff, Jessie began her Evangelist work by lifting up her voice and singing that old favourite, 'The Old Rugged Cross.' She gave it all she had—which was plenty—and, it is recorded by the faithful Press present on the occasion, 'the more orthodox "Amen!" was drowned in secular cheers.'

The sound must have been wine to Jessie—it recalled, no doubt, the resounding huzzas of the Salem court-house—and she warmed to the 8,000 of the faithful.

She spoke in a husky voice, tremulous with emotion.

That is what she said:

'I want to say to-night that I thank God I am saved and that He has brought me back again.'

With that, according to the strict instructions she had received beforehand, she made about to retire. But the crowd would not have it. Again to quote the sprightly Mr Boyer,

> surely it was not the redeemed who rudely shouted the widow's name as her rival fought onwards with the service. There was a miniature sailboat on the stage. The pale-faced Evangelist gestured towards it and one could see her mouth open and shut as she recited her parable. Now and again she tortured her face into a smile, and sometimes phrases sounded through the confusion—"sinking in the sea of sin, sinking to rise no more"—and then at last it was over. Sister Aimée had fought the good fight and it had not been pleasant. Sister Jessie received an ovation as she distributed paperbound copies of the New Testament; when similar scenes happened on succeeding nights, it was unbearable. Mrs Aimée expelled Sister Jessie from her organization, declaring that she had not been sufficiently trained to preach or to make public appearances for the Lord.

The hard-boiled reporters panted for revelations.

'Are you jealous of her?' they asked pertinently.

The reply was as good as could be expected in the difficult circumstances.

'In the Lord's work,' said Aimée Semple MacPherson, 'one is not afraid of a pretty face.' Her own was twisted as she spoke; she might have been eating a sour plum.

That was the end. Released from the Lord's service, Jessie had no further cards to play; she bumped down-hill as though she were descending to Avernus on a rickety toboggan. 'Expelled' by Sister Aimée, it was just as though she was the victim of a curse.

She fought back. She even wrote to President Roosevelt about it, but it was no good; her cup became filled to overflowing; bitterness seeped into her soul.

One must have a certain sympathy with this extraordinary woman. She had been granted a vision of glamour and wealth, and this died hard. She had been told to expect illimitable riches—whereas, all she actually gained was a sum equivalent to £700, plus clothing, furniture, presents and living expenses.

No heroine of maudlin fiction suffered more or so intensely. She became the heroine of Victorian melodrama; she was ejected from her old home—exactly twelve months after her triumphant acquittal. It snowed that day. . . .

In May of the following year, she was forced to ask for relief. She was entitled to do this because her husband had been in the world war, and she was thereby enabled to claim protection under the State Soldiers' Aid Fund. The authorities gave her the exact sum of sixty-five dollars a month, to keep her and her four children.

The end?

My friends, it is a sad one. According to the latest information to hand, our heroine is still alive. But, alas, oblivion has descended upon her in a blue-black cloud. On the afternoon that she received the first instalment of the Soldiers' Aid Grant, she moved with her four children to a five-roomed apartment on the second floor of a two-family house on Ethel Avenue, Peabody. Her rent there was twenty-five dollars a month, and she paid it from her welfare allowance. Is it any wonder that one of her friends recently declared 'that the children might do with a little more clothing, and that food is not too plentiful?'

Jessie is now said to be thin, although there are no grey hairs on that once thickly-thatched black head. Her skin, we are told, is still very white. She can look out of her kitchen window and see her old home just one street away. Perhaps sometimes she thinks of the fireman on his knees—and lying starkly still outside the bathroom.

One might have thought that her spirit would have been broken. Not at all; the same courage that enabled her to face the applauding audiences at her trial now enables her to plan for the future. She has an eye, we are told, on another residence, which could be bought for just over one thousand pounds. She has not the money, but she is hoping that this will turn up.

Perhaps a New Hampshire farmer who knocked at her door one night, his face flushed like a crimson moon, and who said apologetically that 'he hated to bother her, but he wanted to marry her. His wife had died and he was pretty well off,' could have been prevailed upon to provide it—but Jessie said 'No!' For, you see, there was a tag tied to the offer: the New Hampshire farmer naturally wanted a wife who would live with him down on his farm.

Jessie did not see her way to grant such a request. Living in the backwoods was not for her. After all, she had once been a great figure—her name had been in every paper, crowds had cheered wildly every appearance she made. How could she hide herself away in the bleak Middle-West? She turned this farmer down—cold.

The last recorded words of our heroine may or may not be pathetic. When a reporter called upon her concerning the latest offer of marriage, she swept a hand round her present shabby abode and said contemptuously: 'This is only temporary, I shall climb again.'

HAROLD EATON

How Parsimony
Hanged a Poisoner

In the late summer of 1911, Miss Eliza Mary Barrow, an eccentric
spinster of independent means, and a paying-guest at the house of an
insurance-superintendent in Tollington Park, North London, died
after a few days of distressing indisposition.

The doctor who attended the boarder had prescribed the necessary
and usual remedies for epidemic diarrhœa; had done all he could to
treat his patient successfully. But the epidemic prevalent at the time was
severe, and to some extent baffling to the medical profession. Scores of
people were succumbing to its attacks. Therefore, Miss Barrow's
medical advisor was not unduly surprised when his patient was added to
the list of victims. The outcome was unfortunate but unavoidable.

A death certificate was provided showing enteritis, or epidemic
diarrhoea, as the cause of her decease. Miss Barrow was duly buried,
apparently friendless and unmourned, in a cheap public grave, the
reason given for such a course being that there were only a few pounds
left over with which to pay the undertaker's fee.

Shortly after the poverty-stricken burial, however, relatives of the
dead lady inquired into the estate of the deceased, and certain suspicions were awakened which were communicated to the police. As a
result of persistent demands on the part of these relatives, an order to
exhume Miss Barrow's body was obtained, and a post-mortem examination of the remains took place.

The usual secrecy was observed during the exhumation of the body of
the unfortunate Miss Barrow. Behind locked doors the remains of the
spinster were revealed from the coffin reopened by a special undertaker.
The body was abnormally well-preserved, considering that the inter-
ment had taken place some weeks previously, that death had occurred

during hot weather, and that the alleged cause of death had been diarrhœa. All these factors would tend, under ordinary circumstances, towards speedy deterioration of the tissues. Instead, the corpse almost might have been mummified, so complete was its state of preservation.

Such contradiction of pathological fact at once suggested complications in the death of Miss Barrow which fully justified the exhumation. The stomach, stomach-wall, and other organs were placed in special glass jars, duly and firmly sealed, ready for further examination in the laboratory by Dr W.G. Willcox, the world-famous authority on poisons.

The certified cause of death from enteritis or epidemic diarrhœa, inconsistent though it was with the state of the body's appearance some weeks after burial, could not be upset without the deepest investigations. There were, indeed, in Miss Barrow's stomach, definite traces of a natural disease in the form of slightly reddened intestines. But if arsenical poisoning had caused death—and the well-preserved state of the remains immediately gave rise to this terrible suspicion—would it have been apparent to the doctor who had attended the patient for diarrhœa?

Obviously, the local doctor had been entirely satisfied by the results of his observations while attending the patient. That this doctor did not suspect arsenical poisoning was hardly surprising. Even specialists are occasionally puzzled during post-mortem examinations by the arbitrary symptoms of death. An ordinary practitioner would hardly suspect his patient was a victim of aruenical poisoning when her death coincided with a particularly virulent plague of summer diarrhœa—for the symptoms in either case are remarkably similar!

In certain bodies, the behaviour of arsenic is very eccentric; it is indeed one of the trickiest of poisons. There has been at least one case where no traces of the chemical were discovered in a poisoned body! Therefore, even though the presence of arsenic in the exhumed body of Miss Barrow might be unquestioned, this fact did not, by any means, furnish satisfactory proof that actually she had died from the effects of poisoning. Indeed, apparent symptoms of enteritis, as noted upon the death certificate, still lingered in the intestines. These organs certainly were inflamed by diarrhœa. Had Miss Barrow been ill from natural causes? Had the arsenic only contributed towards death, or would the patient have recovered from her diarrhœa had not arsenic been administered? If death, in any case, had been inevitable, a different construction would have been placed upon the circumstances of her decease from that which might at first have been apparent, even if it were proved arsenic had been administered.

It was essential to determine at once the real cause of death. Meanwhile, an indefatigable search was being made amongst the organs of the deceased woman which had been brought away from the mortuary. In turn, the liver, kidneys, intestines, stomach-wall, were examined patiently and scrupulously for the slightest trace of arsenical poisoning. It was found that these reacted to tests for arsenic in such a way that, despite the condition of the intestines, it was decided that epidemic diarrhœa could not have caused death. *Arsenic alone had put the fatal strain upon the heart and brought about the unfortunate spinster's ultimely end.* Medical opinion was that, in her state of health—the dead woman had suffered from asthma and liver disorder—2 grains of the poison would be a fatal dose. Of course, she may have been given more, but it was impossible to tell how much more because, during her illness, her body would reject the poison, to some extent, by vomiting and diarrhœa. Even if she had not suffered from epidemic diarrhœa, there would still have been rejection of the arsenic by natural methods. In other words, she would have had all the symptoms of diarrhœa even if the germ had not been present in her bowels!

The next process in the enquiry was to discover how much arsenic still remained in the body. The famous Marsh test for the presence of arsenic was conducted. Mixing parts of the organs with sulphuric acid, the resultant liquid was treated with reagents until a brown precipitate proved undoubtedly the presence of the poison.

Taking into account the fact that, in the stomach of most people arsenic is usually present in small quantities imbibed through certain foodstuffs—beer and cocoa, for instance, both contain traces of arsenic—analysis found that, apart from the weight of arsenic present in the hair, skin and nails, there were at least 2.01 grains of the poison lingering in the body. Accordingly, through rejection of the arsenic by natural methods, it was calculated that approximately 5 grains of the poison might have been taken two or three days before death. And the opinion generally held was that 2 grains would prove fatal!

There were two points about the death of Miss Barrow which attracted the attention of, and strongly interested the public. Certainly the receipt into Miss Barrow's system of arsenic had been the cause of her death. But even when the presence of arsenic has been proved beyond a shadow of doubt, that fact does not prove that the arsenic was administered maliciously, conversely that it was self-administered, or *when* it was administered!

Considering the third question, an immediate solution was forthcoming. If a moderately large dose of the poison had been given to her, no improvement in Miss Barrow's health just before death would be recorded. Confirmation of this theory came from the doctor who had attended Miss Barrow during her fatal illness. He could report no improvement of the patient's condition during the last three days of her illness.

Thus, a singularly insignificant fact took on a terrible importance. The question—'During what period or periods of her life had arsenic been administered to Miss Barrow?'—was apparently answered.

Reasoning out all the facts, including the report of the analyst, Dr Willcox, it was evident that *arsenic had been administered with fatal results within a period of two or three days before death took place.* Apart from the fact that no improvement had been noted in Miss Barrow's health during the last seventy-two hours of her life, the organs had reacted in such a way as to indicate that before death they had only been recently irritated by the poison. The poisoning from which the dead woman had suffered had been *acute*, i.e. administered in one or two large doses, not *chronic*, i.e. administered in small doses over a long period of time.

Summing up, medical opinion was of the belief that:

(i) One or two large doses of free arsenic had been administered to Miss Barrow.

(ii) They had been administered within a few days of her death.

Working from another angle from the medical investigators, the police had ascertained that certain fly-papers had been purchased by a member of the household in which Miss Barrow had stayed. Here, medicine and police joined hands. Similar fly-papers were procured and experimented upon by Dr W.H. Willcox, Senior Scientific Analyst to the Home Office. An analysis was made of fly-papers which had been purchased at various shops. One contained 3.8 grains of arsenic, another 4.17, another 4.8, and another 6 grains—that was by scientific extraction. Experiments were also conducted to extract arsenic by simply boiling a fly-paper in a little water. It was ascertained that if one were boiled for some minutes nearly all the arsenic came out. When one paper was put in a quarter-pint of water and left standing overnight, it was found that there were 6.6 grains of arsenic in the liquid.

Further, it was discovered that the fluid resulting from boiling of fly-papers would be bitter and the water coloured from the paper. Arsenic solution could be given in meat juice without detection by the patient.

Regarding the amount of arsenic which would be sufficient to kill an adult, experts considered 2.01 grains might prove a fatal dose. Five grains would be fatal.

The story of the Seddon poisoning case is one which, even to-day, more than twenty years after, brings back startling memories of a criminal trial in which a religious-minded insurance inspector and his wife, with the sympathy of over a hundred thousand of their fellow-citizens, jointly fought for their lives.

How they fared; how the husband went to the gallows by the medical evidence given against him; how the wife went free; how the Judge wept, while he passed sentence of death; how every power in the land was moved by Mrs Seddon to free her husband, arraigned on what was said to be the slightest medical evidence ever put forward in a Court of Law, is a real life-story of such poignant drama that it has seldom been equally even in fiction.

But we are not concerned with the picturesqueness of the Court scenes. It is sufficient that we have shown how science, instead of being a matter of scorn, as it had been some years previously, was a most useful ally of criminal investigation, and that, in the future, pathology would play an important part in the discovery of crime. Without medical investigation and its results, the case against Frederick Henry Seddon would never have gone to the jury. As it was, though it could not possibly be proved that Seddon had administered the arsenic, or that arsenic had been derived by him from the fly-papers in question, the case for the Prosecution was very strong indeed. But the difficult task of persuading the jury to accept the scientific version of the crime was yet to begin.

Following the pathological report upon the cause of death of Miss Barrow, the police had discovered motives for the alleged murder. It was found that Seddon benefited directly by the decease of his paying guest, inasmuch as an annuity of £3 per week for life, which he had granted her in exchange for all her worldly possessions, amounting to several thousand pounds capital value, ceased upon her death. Moreover, a considerable sum of liquid cash, in gold and notes, which should have been in the possession of the deceased woman at the time of her death could not be accounted for by the prisoners. Also, notes were traced to have been passed by Mrs Seddon, under an assumed name, and others paid directly into Mr Seddon's banking account. Moreover, the economy exercised by Seddon at Miss Barrow's funeral became a strong link in the evidence against him. *It transpired that he had informed the undertaker that there was only the sum of £4 10s. with which to bury the dead woman, when he knew that to be an absolute untruth.*

A further damning piece of evidence against Seddon was the fact that, though in her will Miss Barrow left her property to her nephew and niece by adoption, no one else was proved to have benefited by her death except Seddon.

Without the essential facts, as laid down by the medical experts, however, there would have been no prosecution at all, despite the suspicion of Miss Barrow's relatives. As it was, if the jury could be satisfied that Miss Barrow had been in the habit of eating arsenic, Frederick Seddon would go scot-free. Even if Seddon's advocate, Mr Edward Marshall Hall, could prove that the arsenic had been administered by some other person over a longer period than that stated by the Prosecution, the case against the prisoner would have been weakened considerably.

Medical evidence alone stood between Seddon and the gallows, and the line of the Defence was to prove weak links in this medical evidence.

Some peculiar facts concerning arsenic and its relation to the human body came to light. Styrian peasants of Hungary are inveterate arsenic-eaters. This vice seldom proves fatal to the peasants. They consume arsenic, gathered from plants, in small quantities over long periods, and their death-rate is not high. Indeed, they live the normal span of life, and often die from natural causes. The state of their bodies after burial is remarkable. They remain in a state of good preservation for many years.

If Miss Barrow then had herself been an arsenic-eater—and it is a fact unknown to many that there were scores of such people in England—or if she had taken arsenic in her medicine some time previous to her death, it was quite possible that, though an autopsy would reveal—as it had done—definite traces of the poison, death might yet have been, as in the case of the Styrians, from natural causes. But 5 grains of arsenic was an exceedingly large quantity of this poison to exist in a body, and logically it could be reasoned that Miss Barrow would have died months previously had she been an arsenic eater, when the poison in her system had accumulated to approximately but 2 grains—a fatal dose, opinion declared.

Mr Marshall Hall, defending Seddon, pointed out that there was no evidence to prove to the contrary that the invalid, ill with diarrhœa, and extremely thirsty, had not drunk accidentally the water in which the fly-papers had been soaked, and which stood in a saucer near the bed.

To support this theory of suicide or death by misadventure, the able advocate reserved a trump-card. 'Why,' he declared scornfully, 'did not Seddon, were he guilty of poisoning Miss Barrow, have the body cremated?' He would have had no difficulty to be sure, in doing this, seeing that the doctor gave a certificate of death from natural causes. Had Miss Barrow been cremated, how could any pathologist have discovered traces of arsenic in her body?

This was an attractive line of thought for the jury. Seddon was being tried upon purely circumstantial evidence, and any suggestion whereby he might have hidden his guilt would appeal to them. Even motive, as the Judge pointed out, was not proof of a crime!

There was nothing circumstantial, however, about the manner in which Miss Barrow had met her death. It had been proved, beyond a doubt, that she had died from arsenical poisoning. The ravages of arsenic in her body had actually been traced. Had not this been proved to the satisfaction of the Prosecution, there was not even a *prima-facie* case to have been made out against Frederick Seddon.

But no one had proved—no one could prove—who had administered the arsenic; yet how could the jury ignore the fact that Seddon's daughter, Margaret, had purchased fly-papers for her parents, and that they had been soaking in water for a few days before Miss Barrow was taken ill?

When the motive of cupidity was considered, the jury had one strong link between medical evidence and the prisoner's charge, against which even the forensic eloquence and shrewd ability of Marshall Hall could not prevail.

The famous advocate voiced his distrust of the Marsh test for arsenic, suggesting that the test was a splendid one for detecting arsenic, but unreliable for the purpose of measuring the quantity taken. He also warned the jury that they must be more than ordinarily careful to remember that the only question with which they were dealing, was— Did the male prisoner, or his wife, acting singly or jointly, administer a fatal dose of arsenic or a series of fatal doses to Miss Barrow between September 2nd and 14th?

In this wise, Marshall Hall tried to discount the evidence of cold science. The jury, the advocate knew, would be impressed by the impartial pathological witnesses whose statements were so difficult to disprove scientifically and therefore scarcely questionable. But Marshall Hall was afraid that the jury might infer that because arsenic had been found in Miss Barrow's body, the only person who could have administered it was Seddon. But the Prosecution never actually put this forward.

With the idea of counteracting the medical evidence and its obvious effect upon the jury, Marshall Hall made splendid capital out of the fact that Seddon had no theoretical or practical knowledge whatever regarding arsenic; was unaware that by boiling down or soaking fly-papers the arsenic would be freed; and that the only reason the fly-papers were introduced into the case was because Miss Barrow had asked that something might be done about the awful summer flies in her bedroom at Tollington Park. She did not want the sticky sort, Marshall Hall pointed out, so arsenious papers were secured to please her. It looked as though, had not arsenious papers been obtained, that Miss Barrow's certificate of death would have remained unchallenged. He believed the arsenic had not come from the fly-papers!

The advocate had himself studied the properties of arsenic in its relation to the human body, and frequently tried to lead witnesses for the Crown into a trap. But he was unsuccessful. He contended that Miss Barrow must have taken arsenic over a longer period than that upon which the prisoners were charged; otherwise, how could the arsenic have reached her hair, when a recent Royal Commission upon the subject of arsenical poisoning had reported amongst its findings that several months must elapse in the case of accumulative dosing of arsenic *before traces were found in the hair!*

This vital point raised by the Defence might easily have freed Seddon but for the minute and careful pathological study made upon Miss Barrow's corpse. Already, laboratory tests had proved that 2.01 grains of arsenic were present in Miss Barrow's body apart from that present in the hair and bones. The estimated amount administered was nearer 5 grains. If, as Marshall Hall pointed out, the arsenic had been administered over a long period in order to reach the hair, how could such a quantity as 5 grains be present in the body at death? Arsenic would have been rejected in the case of a chronic poisoning over the period the advocate suggested, and it was unreasonable to suppose the residue would have gathered to such a quantity as 5 grains before fatal results overtook the woman. Considering the state of her health during the past year, 2.01 grains of arsenic would have been a fatal residue!

Besides, the fly-papers would have produced, when soaked—as undoubtedly they were—about 6 grains of arsenic. What had been done with that 6 grains? They alone had caused death. But the witnesses for the Prosecution said they were satisfied that *the arsenic in the hair had gathered there between the date of death in early September and the exhumation conducted by Dr Spilsbury in November*—i.e. within two months of burial and not during life!

This last piece of evidence was accepted and Seddon's doom was irrevocably sealed. Such medical testimony was far more dangerous to Marshall Hall's cause than all the police evidence collected during the case. Beaten at all points by the cold interpretation of science, another attack was made upon the Prosecution's theory.

'Arsenic,' suggested Marshall Hall, 'was a cure for asthma when taken in certain medicines. This would, no doubt, probably account for the presence of some arsenic in the dead woman's body?'

The jury certainly required proof of this statement. Those who were in sympathy with the prisoner breathed a sigh of relief. After all, he may, even yet, not be found guilty.

But the question proved futile. Medical science once again spoke in favour of the Crown. The medicine that Miss Barrow had taken for her complaint contained such slight traces of arsenic that the poison would have left no appreciable effect upon her body; certainly would not have accumulated sufficiently to have caused either death or ill-health.

Marshall Hall now endeavoured, as a last resort, to suggest to the jury that as arsenic was present in all foodstuffs of a certain kind, its presence would be discovered in an autopsy of almost any person. Would not therefore this fact weigh against the calculations of the medical experts? Especially was this fact important when it was known beyond doubt that the Styrians imbibed arsenic without poisoning effects.

But what was true of the Styrians was not true of an Englishwoman of Miss Barrow's constitution. The theory concerning arsenic in food-stuffs too was dismissed. Foodstuffs did not contain arsenic in quantities sufficient to kill anyone.

The jury found Seddon guilty of murder, while the charge against his wife was not proven, and she was dismissed from the case. Before the verdict was known, however, the interest of hundreds of medical men, and thousands of the general public was aroused. Many medical practitioners thought that the scientific evidence put forward at the trial need not necessarily have convicted Seddon, and instances were given, some true, others supposititious, in which it was sought to prove that many an innocent man could be hanged upon evidence similar to that given by the medical witnesses at the Seddon trial. Arsenic-eaters came forward and gave their own experiences with the hope of saving the prisoner from what they considered to be a miscarriage of justice.

Seddon appealed against his trial. One hundred and fifty thousand signatures were given for his reprieve, including such names as Lord Haddo, Keir Hardie, and George Lansbury. Mr Marshall Hall made another impassioned appeal before Justices Darling, Channell and Coleridge against the jury's verdict.

There was only one line of appeal, and that was to attack the medical evidence. So, with all the forensic eloquence and brilliant reasoning for which he was famed, Marshall Hall endeavoured to explain away the opinions of the pathologist engaged upon the case.

'Granted,' he pointed out, deliberately, 'that arsenic poisoning had caused Miss Barrow's death, that did not prove that Seddon or his wife had administered it.' Continuing, he pointed out that never had a man been convicted on such slender evidence. There was nothing at all to show that Seddon knew the effects of arsenic would give symptoms identical with those of epidemic diarrhœa. Even if there was evidence to prove death was due to arsenical poisoning, there was no proof of Seddon's felonious administration. Forcefully, Marshall Hall drew attention to the fact that only once had the male prisoner given Miss Barrow her medicine, and that was on the evidence of the young boy, Ernest Grant. Was the boy's testimony valuable? It was also pointed out that members of the medical profession were dissatisfied with the medical evidence rendered. Even if Miss Barrow had died from acute arsenical poisoning, the condition of her hair was consistent also with a protracted administration of the poison over some months.

But this latter point had already been determined. After the Judges had retired to consider, Mr Justice Darling informed the advocate that the appeal had been unsuccessful.

In view of the evidence upon which Seddon had been found guilty, tremendous efforts were made to secure his reprieve. Mrs Seddon and her daughter tried to hold a mass meeting in Hyde Park with a view to obtaining signatures for the reprieve. The meeting was broken up in disorder, and Mrs Seddon got away only under police protection.

Seddon was executed in his private clothes, protesting to the last that he was an innocent man.

But for his parsimony in ordering a cheap public burial for his boarder, Miss Barrow, the relatives of the dead woman would probably never have suspected foul play. Seddon had planned an ingenious crime, so much so, that over a hundred thousand people considered him innocent, yet when the plan had succeeded, he made one little slip, namely, economising on the cremation of the body and the funeral of his victim. This little slip cost him life!

JOHN LAWRENCE

The Jekyll and Hyde of New York

Doctor Arthur Warren Waite, dentist and crack tennis player, to all outward seeming was a child of fortune. He had everything the normal man wants and envies in others, good looks, charm of manner, athletic abilities, a charming wife, and a millionaire father-in-law.

Let us particularize. In appearance Doctor Waite was the typical athletic American, clean-shaven, clear-eyed, regular-featured and frankly healthy. He was popular with men and women alike, and all with whom he came in contact trusted him. He was always perfectly groomed and had that *savoir faire* which comes from wide travel. A witty conversationalist, he could talk entertainingly on most subjects, and he was much in demand by the hostesses of New York.

His father-in-law was John E. Peck, a retired millionaire druggist of Grand Rapids, Michigan, of which town Waite himself was a native. Waite's parents were not well-to-do, but their son showed such brilliance and promise that he was encouraged in every possible way to obtain the best education which they could afford. He went to the University of Michigan and there took a dental course.

From there the brilliant student went to London and afterwards to South Africa, where he did a certain amount of practice in the profession for which he had been trained. Shortly after the outbreak of the Great War he returned to the United States and to his native town. There he met Miss Clara Peck. In spite of the wide gulf between their financial positions, a gulf which might almost have made people suspect he was a fortune hunter, no suggestion of the kind was made when it became known that the two were engaged. Everyone who met the good-looking dentist predicted such a successful career for him that he would never be in any financial difficulties.

Clara Peck and Arthur Warren Waite were married at Grand Rapids in September, 1915. To the surprise of many, however, he did not begin practising there, but moved at once to New York on the plea that the opportunities for advancement were much greater in that town, and his newly-married wife would have greater chances of amusement.

Waite was in no hurry to begin practising. He had always shown a great interest in medicine, and within a few days of arriving in New York he had got in touch with a number of doctors whom he deluded into believing he was a fully-qualified man himself, wealthy, and interested in scientific research, especially the study of bacteriology.

A certain amount of verisimilitude was given to Waite's story by the fact that he had a flat in the exclusive Riverside Drive Apartments, a flat which was richly furnished. The doctor was also well-known as a very good amateur tennis player who had only recently taken part in a number of tournaments at Palm Beach, Florida. He had, too, a considerable amount of medical knowledge, partly acquired through his study of dentistry, and partly learnt through an instinctive desire to acquire knowledge which might prove of use to him in later years.

Through various influences Waite got in touch with Dr Percival L. de Nyce, who was in charge of the bacteriological laboratory of the Flower Hospital, one of the best known institutions in New York. Dr Nyce was impressed with his new pupil, and the extraordinarily keen interest he took in all germ cultures. But it was only in the most virulent and deadly germs that his pupil was really interested, and he actually complained to Dr Nyce that the germs he was studying were not virulent enough for the experiments he had in mind!

Clara Waite firmly believed her husband was in practice as a doctor, and once or twice, in order to foster that belief and account for the necessary income to keep up their expensive style of living, he took her to the Flower Hospital and asked her to stay in the waiting room for a while. After keeping her there kicking her heels for half an hour or so, and reflecting on what he might be doing, he would return and announce that he had just finished an important operation. The deluded Clara, who understood not a single detail of the medical account her husband gave her, was full of pride that his abilities were being recognised in such an important institution.

It may well be asked at this stage, where was the comparatively poor student of a year or two ago getting the large sums of money which were necessary not only for his living expenses but for those in connection with the bacteriological experiments he was carrying out?

Waite had ingratiated himself so well with the Peck family that, with one exception, they were intensely proud of the brilliant addition to it. His wife's father helped financially so that his son-in-law should not be handicapped in any of his research work which he represented was necessary to advance in his profession. He not only gave his daughter a very handsome dowry, out of which the Riverside apartments were so luxuriously furnished, but he allowed her £60 a month.

It must be admitted that Waite had an exceedingly great attraction for women, especially for women older than himself. Mrs Peck adored him. Nothing he could do was wrong, and her sister-in-law, Miss Catherine Peck, who had given her niece a cheque for nearly a thousand pounds as a wedding present, had even a higher opinion of him. So much did she value his advice, indeed, that she was easily persuaded to let him have £10,000 of her money to invest. It was on this money that Waite lived. Aunt Catherine was unwise enough to let it be known that on her death Waite would receive a very substantial legacy. It was also common knowledge in the family that Mr Peck's will left half his fortune to his daughter Clara. If Mr and Mrs Peck died, and Aunt Catherine died, and perhaps later on Clara Waite, Arthur Warren Waite would be a very rich and eligible widower!

A few weeks after their arrival in New York the devoted young husband—and there was not the slightest doubt that to all outward appearances he was infatuated with his young wife—suggested that her mother and father should be asked to stay with them for a while. Both parents were delighted to accept their son-in-law's invitation, but neither stayed very long on this first visit, for the air of New York did not seem to agree with Mr Peck. He felt run down almost as soon as he arrived. His son-in-law diagnosed a coming cold and sprayed his throat every evening. But that did not ward off the feeling of lassitude, any more than did the medicine which Waite had made up, and Mr Peck returned to Grand Rapids to be thoroughly overhauled there by his own doctors. They confessed themselves completely puzzled. However the air of Grand Rapids certainly suited old Mr Peck better than did that of New York and he was soon feeling as fit as ever.

Mrs Peck had found the visit to her beloved daughter and son-in-law all too short and as soon as she was satisfied that her husband was on the road to recovery and not likely to have a relapse, she paid them another visit—her last. Shortly after her arrival, she, too, began to feel ill, and a

Doctor Porter was called in. He diagnosed that there was nothing very much the matter, though Dr Waite strongly disagreed, and asserted that he was sure his mother-in-law was seriously ill.

One night when Dr Waite was out ostensibly visiting his patients, a very remarkable incident occurred, though no one thought much about it at the time. Mrs Waite, who had gone to bed, detected a strong smell of gas and traced it as coming from her mother's room. When she entered it she found that the tap of the gas stove had been left on and if it had not been for the fact one of the windows was partly open there is no doubt her mother would have been asphyxiated.

From that day, however, Mrs Peck grew steadily worse, and on January 30th, 1916, she died. Doctor Porter, who had suspected nothing wrong, readily gave his certificate. Dr Waite, who seemed utterly grief-stricken by his mother-in-law's sudden death, accompanied her body to Grand Rapids, where he told various members of the family that her last dying wish was that she should be cremated. The ashes were buried in the family vault. The act of cremation had effectively destroyed all danger of anyone finding out the real cause of the old lady's death.

Mr Peck was overwhelmed by the loss of his wife and in February he accepted a second invitation to come to New York to visit his daughter. Both he and Clara had been very fond of Mrs Peck and both were eager to be together in their common sorrow. Old Mr Peck, too, liked his son-in-law, for the latter had been more sympathetic than even a devoted son-in-law might be expected to be. Waite was so charming, so anxious to make his father-in-law forget, so full of warmth on the old man's arrival, that for a few days Mr Peck really was cheered up and felt far less lonely than he had been feeling since his wife's death. There was a very strong bond of affection between his daughter and himself, for in her he saw again the mother as she was in the days when he first courted her and began his successful struggle for fortune.

During those early days of Mr Peck's second visit to the Riverside Apartment there occurred an incident which has a considerable bearing on the rest of the story. Dr Waite, as far as his devoted wife Clara knew, and her father knew, was an exceedingly busy man. He had to be out many evenings visiting his patients, and sometimes he was so hard-pressed that he did not return until the early hours of the morning. Actually Waite was very fond of wine, women and song. He had early discovered that he exercised a peculiar influence over women, and his life in New York was a continual round of gaiety. Although the delightful doctor distributed his favours on a fairly lavish scale, entertaining at the most expensive restaurants and dance cafés those whom he favoured, there was one lady in particular who proved more attractive than the rest, a Mrs Horton.

Margaret Horton, a beautiful young grass widow, had met Waite first at the Berlitz School of Languages. She was ambitious to become an opera singer. In a few days Waite had installed her in a suite of rooms at the Hotel Plaza. He himself was very fond of music and the two proved very congenial company for one another.

'Dr Waite had an extraordinary kind heart,' she said some months after their first meeting. 'He loved all the fine sentiments and the beautiful things of life. He used to say to me, 'Margaret, when you sing you make me weep, because you make me think of beautiful things'. He loved music. It was that love of music which drew us together.'

It was while dining with Margaret Horton that Waite was seen by a Doctor Cornell, a relative of the Peck family, and a Miss Hardwicke. When Waite saw Cornell he made an excuse to his companion and walked across to the other table. He explained glibly that he had just completed an important operation.

'I have brought my own special nurse with me for dinner as I felt that she deserved something out of the ordinary for her skill and devotion to my work,' he explained.

He told his story with easy confidence and all those at the table, with the exception of Miss Hardwicke, were inclined to believe it. But she had been watching Waite and Margaret Horton, and she was secretly convinced that there was a deeper relationship between the two than that of doctor and nurse. But she made no outward comment, though the time was soon to come when she was to crystallize her suspicions into such drastic action that Waite's name, in consequence, was to fill the front pages of the American newspapers for many a long day.

A few days after the incident in the restaurant Mr Peck was taken seriously ill and a Dr Moore was called in. He diagnosed digestive trouble and prescribed accordingly. Mr Peck's son-in-law was most attentive. The sick man did not like his medicine and Dr Waite soon found a way out of the difficulty. One evening Waite came into the kitchen and without any disguise poured some medicine into his father-in-law's soup. Later in the evening he came into the kitchen again when tea was being prepared for Mr Peck and poured some further medicine into the teapot.

'Dora,' he explained to the servant, 'father didn't like his soup, so I must put some more medicine in his tea.'

Although Dr Moore had not considered the condition of his patient to be very serious, Dr Waite, as in the case of Mrs Peck, disagreed with him.

'He hasn't a very strong constitution,' he declared, 'and I should not be surprised if he did not live for long.'

As with Mrs Peck, Waite's prophecy proved more accurate than had that of other doctors. On March 12th, but six weeks after his wife's death, Mr Peck died, and Clara Waite had lost both her parents. And as with the case of Mrs Peck, Waite declared that his father-in-law's last wish was that he should be cremated and his ashes placed beside those of his wife. Accordingly, the body, accompanied by the grief-stricken Clara and her sorrowing husband, was taken to Grand Rapids for that purpose. Before that journey, however, the body had been embalmed, a fact which should be borne in mind.

To Dr Waite's astonishment he found when he got to Grand Rapids that the family were not in favour of the old man being cremated. He was careful enough, however, not to raise any great objections, and after duly seeing his father-in-law buried he hurried back to New York—and Mrs Horton. Of late he had been spending money freely, too freely, but now, under his father-in-law's will, through Clara, he would have no cause to worry about money for some time. When he had, there was always Miss Catherine Peck, who had promised him a substantial legacy on her death.

There was one member of the Peck family who had never been very friendly with Dr Waite, who had always disliked him in fact, despite his great charm. That was Percival Peck, Clara's only brother. It was Percival Peck who had raised the greatest objections to his father being cremated. Just before the arrival of the body at Grand Rapids he had received a mysterious telegram from New York which read as follows:

'Suspicions aroused. Demand autopsy. Keep telegram secret.—K. Adams.'

The name of Adams was quite unknown to Percival Peck, but that fact did not influence him in the least. It transpired afterwards that K. Adams was the Miss Hardwicke who had seen Dr Waite and Mrs

Horton dining together, and who had disbelieved the story the former told that the lady was his nurse. But the telegram, from whatever source it came, provided young Peck with an opportunity which he eagerly seized. He had a secret examination made of his father's body and at the same time employed private detectives to keep an eye on his brother-in-law and keep a record of his movements.

Clara, who had become seriously ill following upon the double shock of her mother's and father's deaths, had stayed behind at Grand Rapids, while her husband had hurried back to the gaities of New York.

And then Waite received his first shock. He had left Grand Rapids fully satisfied that he had bluffed everyone, that he could now spend money just as freely as he wished, enjoy himself to the top of his bent. But a few days after his return Mr Peck's son-in-law received a shock. The undertaker who had arranged for the embalming of Mr Peck called upon him and asked that his bill should be paid.

'What's the hurry?' asked Waite. 'You know the money is safe enough, don't you?'

He was surprised at the sudden demand for the bill, but he was more than surprised by the undertaker's reply. It worried him. It was the tiny black cloud on the edge of the horizon.

'It's really Mr Kane, sir, the embalmer,' explained the undertaker. 'He thinks he might not get his money.'

'Why?' demanded Waite, struck by the uneasy look in the other's face.

'Well, there's some idea that arsenic had been used,' explained the undertaker.

Waite was well aware that it was against the law for arsenic to be used in any embalming fluid, as he was also aware that arsenic would be found in Mr Peck's body if it were examined.

'I think I'd better see Mr Kane,' he said evenly.

When the doctor saw Kane he did not beat about the bush.

'How much is it worth to you to say that you used arsenic?' he asked.

The embalmer named a sum, and after some haggling Waite agreed to pay him $9,000. But Kane's nerve broke at the last minute and he told a remarkable story to the police when questioned.

'Waite told me he was in a hole and asked me to put arsenic in the sample of embalming fluid I was to give the District Attorney. He said he would make me independent for life if I did what I was asked.'

Waite by now suspected that his movements were being watched and he arranged for Kane to meet him casually in a cigar store.

'I met him there by a telephone booth,' Kane related. 'And he gave me a big roll of bills. I was so scared that I could hardly tell where I was. I stood there with the money in my hand.

' "For God's sake get that stuff out of sight," Dr Waite said, "and get the sample down to the District Attorney's office."

'I went right home; I was so nervous that I couldn't count the money. I tried afterwards and couldn't do it. I put it in a bureau drawer. I was so nervous about the money that my wife noticed it. She got to worrying me and at last made me go to a doctor to find out if I was sick. I knew all right, but I didn't tell her. I shook like a leaf every now and then when I got to thinking about the money in the bureau drawer. Then I took it down to Greenport and buried it. I didn't put anything into the sample of my embalming fluid. I made up the sample just as I always make the fluid.'

Kane's own record wasn't of the best. He had been suspected on more than one occasion of helping clients 'who were in a hole' out of it on the payment of a reasonably large sum. But for the fact that Percival Peck had brought pressure to bear with the authorities and had had his own private detectives following his brother-in-law, the interview between Kane and Waite and the handing over of a large sum of money in the cigar store might not have been known until too late. But within a very short time of the meeting, it had been reported to the police, and Kane was asked for the sample of his fluid. Rumours were flying about, and it was these rumours coming to his ears which made him break down. He had embalmed the body of Mr Peck before it had been conveyed to Grand Rapids and he was now beginning to realize that there was trouble ahead. And this wouldn't be the first time he had been in trouble.

The District Attorney's suspicions had been aroused on receiving a report from Professor Vaughan, of the University of Michigan, who had made an examination of Mr Peck's body. He had sent in a report to the effect that the millionaire had died from arsenic poisoning. There was just a possibility that the arsenic had been in the embalming fluid, but when he heard Kane's story he immediately issued a warrant for the arrest of Waite.

The iron nerve of the suspected man was breaking fast under the strain of waiting, and it broke a few hours before the detectives called at his Riverside Apartments with the warrant for his arrest. He was found unconscious in the room adjoining that in which Mr and Mrs Peck had died.

But Waite was not to evade the law so easily. He was rushed to the hospital and strong emetics administered. In the hands of skilful physicians he made a rapid recovery. While he was getting over the effect of the drugs he had taken, however, he was thinking out what story to tell. He was now fully aware of the likely evidence against him and only a miracle could save him. He decided to play the part of Dr Jekyll and Mr Hyde.

When questioned by the District Attorney in hospital Waite at once admitted that he had given his father-in-law arsenic.

'Have you any accomplices?'

'Only this other fellow,' replied the accused man with elaborate carelessness.

'What other fellow?'

'The man from Egypt. He's always been inside me ever since I can remember. He has made me do things against my will. He made me take up the study of germs, as if I used them I wouldn't be detected. I was compelled against my will to put them in my father-in-law's food. Try as I would I could not get rid of my murderous other self. Often I have gone for long walks and fought against the evil one, and tried to run away from him. But he was so fleet of foot that he always caught me up.'

So earnestly did Waite tell his story that it was partly believed.

'Did this Egyptian make you kill Mr Peck?' he was asked.

'When my father-in-law came to stay with us I wanted to help him all I could. Then the man from Egypt said Mr Peck was too old to live, that he ought to die, and if he did die I wouldn't have to worry about money. He brushed aside all my arguments. When Mr Peck had first visited us the Egyptian made me spray his throat with germs, but though they made him ill they did not kill him. I was ordered this time to use arsenic as it was quicker. I was told to put it in his soup and tea and egg nog. I did my best, but the Egyptian was in control. Try as I could I found it impossible to get rid of him. But now that he has forced me to do these things he has left me, and for the first time I felt that my soul is free. He seemed to leave me last night and he hasn't returned again to-day to torture me with his evil suggestions.'

The story told by Waite had exactly the effect he foresaw. It was so wild that it seemed as though only a madman could tell it. Some of the leading alienists in America were called in by the prosecution as well as by the defence.

Dr Jeliffe, the leading alienist for the prosecution, said at the trial, 'In my opinion the prisoner was sane and knew the nature and quality of his act. He was fully aware of all the phases of his crime. In my opinion he is an average man, somewhat superficial, inclined to be snobbish and of no great intellectual attainments.'

With that a number of other leading doctors agreed and ultimately their opinion prevailed.

While he was waiting his trial an amazing story came to light. Some of this has already been told. A search of Waite's flat resulted in the discovery of a number of books on poisons and a hundred and eighty slides containing germs of tetanus (lockjaw), typhoid, diphtheria, cholera and other deadly diseases with which he had been experimenting. He had spent large sums on women and amusement and had given Mrs Horton jewellery which had been entrusted to him by Miss Catherine Peck. Practically all the money the latter had given him to invest had gone in riotous living. Only the death of his father-in-law, indeed, could save him from exposure and ruin. So cunningly had he disguised his various amours that until he was arrested his wife had no knowledge of them.

'I was so shocked and amazed that I could not believe them true,' she declared after her husband's arrest. 'It seems impossible that a man who has been so uniformly gentle and kind to me and apparently so loyal could be guilty of the crime with which he is charged.'

Dozens of people who knew Waite well were as puzzled. Many believed that he really was a Jekyll and Hyde, that he had been obsessed by the man from Egypt, as he asserted. Others asserted that the story was told deliberately in an attempt to evade the law. There was one man who never believed for one single moment that the doctor was insane. That was Percival Peck, the man who had received the mysterious telegram and acted on it so promptly, the man who at once employed private detectives to follow his brother-in-law's movements, who never ceased his efforts to unearth everything he could to prove Waite's guilt.

'I know that Arthur is guilty,' he declared shortly after Waite's arrest. 'The electric chair will be too good for him. Even if he were tortured his death would never bring back my beloved parents or pay for his horrible deeds. I will do all in my power to see that he is found guilty and executed.

'He is surely entitled to no consideration whatever. I am convinced that Dr Waite married my sister Clara with but one idea, and that was to get her money. Even before her mother died he predicted an untimely death for us all. We believed him to be a surgeon, and when mother died we suspected nothing. Even when the news of father's death came we did not suspect until I got that telegram. I am sure if it had not been for that my sister and my aunt would have died next.'

Percival Peck was adamant to the last. He approached the prosecution shortly before the trial and said:

'I have only one favour to ask, and that is that I have a seat through every minute of the trial near that man, so that I can see the last gleam of hope gradually fade from his face.'

In the witness-box Waite was perfectly cool, and he made no attempt to hide the appallingly evil personality of the man from Egypt who had compelled him to commit and contemplate crimes which shocked even New York. The more terrible his story, the more coolly it was told, the greater the chance the jury would believe that only a madman could do these things. His own counsel, by clever questions, brought out details of the murder of Mrs Peck and her husband which seemed to show that only a madman could have acted the way Waite did.

'What did you do after you had given your mother-in-law the fatal dose of poison?' asked his counsel.

'Why, I went to sleep, of course,' answered the prisoner in the witness-box. He added that in the morning he went along to his mother-in-law's bedroom and, finding her dead, quietly came out of the room again and waited for his wife to make the discovery her mother had died in the night. He told the jury of all the ways he had afterwards tried to kill Mr Peck before he finally succeeded.

'I gave him a throat spray and a nasal spray containing germs, and when that didn't work I got a lot of calomel which I administered to him in order to weaken him so that he could not resist the germs, but it failed. The man recovered every time. I would get him to go out and expose himself to draughts in the hope that he would catch cold, and I dampened his sheets for the same reason. Once I got some hyrochloric acid and put in the radiator in his room expecting the fumes would affect him. Finally I gave him arsenic. I sat up with him that night, as my wife was tired. He was in great pain, groaning. I gave him some chloroform and when he was unconscious I placed a pillow over his face and kept it there until he died.'

Is that evidence of a sane man or not?

'Waite has told you the truth. There is no part of his story that is not true,' said the counsel for the defence in his final speech. 'He has no moral sense whatever. What are we going to do with such a man as this? You would not sent to the electric chair an idiot, a lunatic or a child. On the other hand we cannot permit such a man as Waite to be at large. We must remove him from society by placing him in an institution.'

Mr Justice Shearn demolished the arguments of the counsel for the defence, in his address to the jury.

'You are not concerned at all with the question of the punishment of this man. The question raised by defendant's counsel of what to do with such a man is not the question at all. The law determines what shall be done. Your function is to determine the facts so that the law may operate.

'Don't get into your heads that you are called upon to determine anything but the facts. Juries have no right to set up standards of what constitutes right and wrong, and no right to discuss how the law shall deal with a man like this. You must not attempt to usurp the function of the Legislature.

'In this case no claim is made that the defendant did it in the heat of passion. On the contrary he himself admits premeditation, intent and a motive. No matter what the defendant has confessed you must remember the burden still rests upon the prosecution to establish his guilt beyond a reasonable doubt. The defendant is entitled to have the case determined on the facts and not on what he says.'

Part of the remainder of the judge's summing up is so phrased that a copy of it should be handed to every jury in a murder case where the defence is one of insanity.

'You might infer from arguments of counsel and some of the evidence that you are here to hold a medical clinic. That's not so at all. It would be absurd to ask twelve laymen to determine whether from the medical point of view a man is sane or insane, especially as men learned in the profession do not agree on the matter. The question is not whether he is sane but whether he was responsible under the tests prescribed by the law—that is, did he know the nature and quality of the act and know it was wrong. That's not a test for experts, but for men of commonsense. Moral indifference is not insanity.

'The claim that the defendant was weak in will power and that he was unable to resist suggestions like those from 'the Man from Egypt' has also been passed on by the highest courts, who have held that, no matter what medical authority there may be for such a claim, it cannot be assented to by the courts. Indulgence in evil passions weakens the will power and at the same time the sense of responsibility.'

The trial was very much shorter than the great majority of sensational murder trials in America, where money can hold up justice for months. The trial only took five days and the jury were only a little over an hour bringing in their verdict of 'Guilty.'

To the last the condemned man showed that curious double personality which puzzled all those with whom he came in contact. He never wearied of talking about himself.

'My life consisted of lying, cheating, stealing and killing. My personality was that of a gentleman and I went for music, art and poetry.'

He dedicated a long poem to himself, an address to his body by his soul after death.

> 'And thou are dead, dear comrade,
> In whom I dwelt a time,
> With whom I strolled through star-kissed bowers
> Of fragrant jessamine.
> And thou wert weak, O comrade,
> Thyself in self did fail,
> And now the stars are turned to tears
> and sobs the nightingale.
> And though I now must leave you,
> The same old songs I'll sing,
> And o'er yon hill the same soft dew
> Will spread its silver wing.
> Across the fields, among the stars,
> I now must go alone,
> Your spirit now will roam afar,
> And leave you, friend, alone.'

A few days before his execution, when he was reading the Bible, he remarked with his usual charming smile, 'I was looking over the ten Commandments and found I had broken all but one—the one about profanity. I have never been profane.'

He kept up his story about his two personalities until the last.

But it did not save him. He went to his death with that boyish smile and charming manner which had characterised him from the day he began his career.

ALAN HYND

The Case of the Lady Who Lost her Head

When, in 1889, Miss Kunigunde Mackamotzki of Brooklyn decided, at the age of seventeen, to change her name to Cora Turner she touched off a chain reaction that was to have far-reaching consequences. Miss Mackamotzki had found that her family name, of Polish origin, acted as a layer of insulation between her and gainful employment. Prospective employers had gagged at the thought of being obliged to pronounce either the girl's first name or her last one several times a day. She had hardly begun to call herself Cora Turner when a Brooklyn physician took her on as a secretary.

Had Kunigunde Mackamotzki not changed her name she would not have secured the position with the physician and had she not secured the position she would not have come under the brooding scrutiny of one of her employer's professional colleagues. This colleague was an unobstrusive, undersized widower of thirty-one named Dr Hawley Harvey Crippen. Dr Crippen, who was obliged to wear thick-lensed glasses because of an affliction that caused him constantly to blink his bulging blue eyes, was, of all things, an eye specialist. He shared offices with Cora Turner's employer and one day, shortly after she had first gone to work for the doctor, Cora got a speck of something in her eye and availed herself of the professional services of Dr Crippen.

Although Cora was only seventeen, she had what it took to make the eye specialist forget, for the very first time, the wife who had died of tuberculosis about a year previously. The girl, an olive-skinned brunette, was over-developed in the right places and gave off strong and unmistakable cosmic vibrations. Dr Crippen tried to seduce her, but she was for sale, not for rent. She hooked him, three months after he took the speck out of her eye, for a marriage certificate.

189

The Crippens took up housekeeping in the remote reaches of Brooklyn and then there came, as William Bendix would say, a revolting development. Cora Crippen had vocal aspirations. She practiced scales without regard to the hour of day or night. Her voice—a thin soprano—wasn't good, but it wasn't exactly bad, either. That, as it was to turn out, was just the trouble. Had Cora Crippen's voice been better than it was, or worse, or had her father been President, a decision as to what to do with it, one way or the other, could eventually have been reached. 'You never told me you sang,' Dr Crippen said to his bride one night, when, after a long day of peering into eyeballs, he was hardly in a mood to whip up enthusiasm for his wife's flights up and down the octaves. Cora struck a dramatic pose. 'I wanted to surprise you,' she said. 'I am going to be a great opera star.'

As time went on, the eye doctor found himself astride a two-horned dilemma, one horn being music, the other—let's face it—sex. The former Kunigunde Mackamotzki turned out to be the kind of girl who might today be referred to, in a certain California community that shall be nameless, as an oversexed nymphomaniac. That was fine with the little eye doctor. The trouble was that if Crippen loved his wife he had to love her voice too. He decided to do all he could to further Cora's musical ambitions; the thought never entered his head that the Polish girl, accommodating as she was, looked upon him privately as an important rung on the ladder of ambition.

Dr Crippen soon found his pockets being turned inside out by vocal coaches and theatrical agents who promised to do great things for his wife. The young lady herself was so certain that she would eventually be on a competitive basis with Adelina Patti and Madam Melba that she even chose a professional name. She began calling herself Belle Elmore. After a couple of years of horsing around with teachers and agents, and his wife getting nowhere, Dr Crippen, whose practice had never been very good, found himself being practically blown face downward by panting creditors immediately to the rear. Although he realized that Cora was responsible for his plight, the thought of remonstrating with her, let alone leaving her, never visited him. Life without her was unthinkable.

Crippen wangled a job as medical expert for a patent-medicine outfit in St Louis. As a native of Coldwater, Michigan, he knew and liked the Middle West; he figured that the down-to-earth climate of Missouri would cause his wife's ambition to wither and die.

Nothing of the sort happened. Cora Crippen dug up not only swindling vocal coaches and grasping agents in St Louis, but expensive costumiers who catered to the ham in her by decking her out like Aïda and other operatic heroines. Dr Crippen eventually found himself as deep in the financial mire of St Louis as he had been in Brooklyn and was obliged to shift his base of operations. He practiced successively in Toronto, Salt Lake City and Philadelphia, but always the end was the same—his wife's ambition to become a singer used up money faster than he could make it.

In 1900—the eleventh year of his marriage—Dr Crippen, at the age of forty-two, looked like a well-preserved fifty-five. The financial strain of life during the day, and the glandular demands of life at night, had made him an old man before his time. His sandy moustache was now flecked with gray, and his forehead had begun a retreat. Cora Crippen, now twenty-eight, had yet to appear on a stage; she had, moreover, begun to show the first signs of frustration. She began to quarrel with Crippen, find fault with him and, perish the thought, lock the bedroom door on him.

When Crippen got the chance to go to London as a salesman for Munyon's Remedies, another patent-medicine outfit, he grabbed it. He thought a change of countries might put his relationship with Cora back where it had once been. The Crippens took rooms in Bloomsbury. While Dr Crippen was out peddling nostrums, his wife began to hang around the offices of music-hall agents. Belle Elmore, as Mrs Crippen was still calling herself, had lowered her sights a little; if she couldn't make Covent Garden she would settle for the variety stage. Thus the whole cruel wheel started to roll again.

Six years passed. In 1906, Dr Crippen, making out well enough with the Munyon people to achieve a Mexican stand-off with the wolf at the door, rented a little semi-detached torture chamber in Hilldrop Crescent, a quiet, leafy thoroughfare off the Camden Road in the Holloway district. Cora Crippen had by this time become acquainted with several broken-down actors and actresses. She invited the Thespians to the house for parties at night and on Saturday afternoons and Sundays—anything to maintain contact with the theatre. Dr Crippen had little difficulty in churning up an active dislike for his wife's closest friend—a variety actress named Lil Hawthorne. Miss Hawthorne was a brassy character of middle age with a strong affinity for other people's business; the doctor couldn't dislodge the feeling that she was collaborating with his wife in hollowing out a tunnel under him.

Cora Croppen's parties took money. Crippen often asked himself why he paid for food and liquor for his wife's friends; he didn't seem to realize it, but he was chasing something that had long since vanished. His wife had become more disagreeable to him than ever. Her deepening frustration had driven her to the compensations of starches, fats and sweets and these in turn had obscured her once exciting contours.

Crippen, now definitely a fifth wheel on a wagon but quiet and uncomplaining, fixed up a little den for himself in the attic of the house. When, of a night or a Saturday afternoon, he would get off a tram on the Camden Road and swing into Hilldrop Crescent, weary from plowing the patent-medicine field, and hear the merry sounds of another of his wife's parties, he would slip into the house the back way, grab something from the kitchen, tip-toe up to the attic, and lock himself in his den. To fill in the lonely hours he took up light reading and became interested in the works of William LeQueux, an English mystery novelist.

LeQueux had, while prowling a second-hand book store in Stockholm, come upon a rare book, published in Petrograd in 1869, entitled *Secrets of the States of Venice*. The volume, printed in Latin and old Italian, both of which LeQueux understood, gave detailed formulas for the slow, lethal and undetectable poisons by which upper-class Venetians abbreviated associations with enemies, friends and chance acquaintances. In one of his novels, LeQueux made casual reference to *Secrets of the States of Venice*, mentioning that the volume detailed the formulas for ancient, undetectable poisons without dwelling on the formulas themselves.

When Dr Crippen, reading LeQueux in his attic retreat, came upon the reference to the rare old book, his professional curiosity was piqued. Having been grounded in the basic poisons during his studies at the Hospital College in Cleveland and at Ophthalmic Hospital in New York, the doctor wondered what the Venetians had had that modern poisoners did not have. Was it possible that the rare book to which LeQueux referred contained the key to some long-lost knowledge that the medical profession could put to advantage—or, more to the point, knowledge that Dr Crippen himself, ever on the qui vive for a stray pound, could monetize?

Crippen began to spend his spare time in the second-hand book stalls, trying to track down a copy of *Secrets of the States of Venice*. Failing to locate the book, he wrote to LeQueux, in March of 1908, for an appointment. For some reason or other, perhaps so that his motives wouldn't be misunderstood, Dr Crippen used the name of Dr Adams in writing to the author. LeQueux made an appointment for Dr Adams to have some Scotch and soda with him at the Devonshire Club. Crippen opened the conservation by saying that he liked LeQueux's mysteries even better than those of Conan Doyle—a remark that didn't exactly offend the author—and then got around to the subject of poisons. He wondered if Le Queux might be so kind as to lead him to the whereabouts of that copy of *Secrets of the States of Venice* so casually mentioned in one of his books. LeQueux said he would be happy to oblige but the book was in storage in Italy. Crippen seemed deeply disappointed. 'Well,' he said, 'can you tell me anything about those formulas that are in that book—those formulas for poisons that left not the slightest trace?' LeQueux recalled that the volume had mentioned several such poisons, but of course he didn't remember sufficient details to deal them off the cuff now. Anyway, he doubted that many of the so-called undetectable poisons of ancient Venice would be quite so undetectable if subjected to modern toxicological analysis.

Mrs Crippen's good friend, Lil Hawthorne, the variety actress, had been instrumental in obtaining for her the job as treasurer of the Music Hall Ladies' Guild, a charitable organization for indigent female Thespians. The post, part-time and no pay, broadened Mrs Crippen's theatrical contacts and her parties took on proportionate stature.

In September of 1908, six months after he had met LeQueux, Crippen landed a couple of extra part-time jobs—one with an ear-trumpet concern, the other with a dental company that manufactured false teeth on an assembly-belt basis. The arrangement was that he was to sell the products of both outfits, on a commission basis, but that the jobs were not to interfere with his main employment with Munyon's Remedies. The dental concern was a large and prominent organization with offices in Albion House, New Oxford Street, and Crippen, although employed only part time and on a commission basis, found that he had a secretary at his disposal.

The secretary was a dark, tiny and moderately attractive young lady bearing the somewhat improbable name of Ethel LeNeve. She was on the self-effacing side, but it was this very quality, contrasted to Cora Crippen's drum-majorette approach to life, that first attracted Dr Crippen to her. Because of Ethel LeNeve, Dr Hawley Harvey Crippen saw Cora Crippen, clearly and for the very first time, for what she had become—a fat, faded, frustrated woman who, although only thirty-six, looked to be in her middle forties.

Dr Crippen and his secretary—she twenty-five, he fifty—quickly became clandestine lovers. From all accounts, the little man was passing through that biological stage that today is recognized as the male menopause. He was flattered and exhilarated, and endowed with a new confidence in himself, because he could attract and hold a girl half his age. As for the girl, she was complimented by the attentions of an older man whose education and manners were in sharp contrast to those of the plumbers' apprentices she had known in the Provinces before coming to London.

Ethel LeNeve had lodgings not far from Albion House and Crippen spent many a night there, telling his wife that he had to go out of town on business. When he did spend an evening at Hilldrop Crescent, it was in the attic, locked in his den. The relationship between the Crippens now resembled an armed truce.

Crippen's affair with Miss LeNeve, like his wife's parties, took money, and business in the three lines he was in was not so good. The patent-medicine game was off; the dental field was depressed because people were making their old choppers, or their gums, do instead of investing in new false teeth; and the ear-trumpet market was scraping a new low, perhaps because the everyday news in the Britain of 1908 was approximately as hilarious as it is today and people who were hard of hearing got wise to the fact that they were, in a way, well off.

Crippen decided he might pick up some extra money by contriving a plot for a mystery story and selling it to LeQueux. He immersed himself in volumes on poisons. He read practically everything that was in print on the subject of toxicology; he became an authority on the Manual of Dr Rudolph August Witthaus, the American toxicologist whose conclusions were being generally accepted as standard, particularly at murder trials. Crippen, still calling himself Dr Adams, saw LeQueux several times late in 1908 and early in 1909. At each meeting, the little doctor had a plot for the novelist that turned on a murder by poison. The basic plot was always the same: A man poisoned his wife, secreted her body, and ran off with a mistress. The man in the Crippen plot always got away with murder so that the plot had, from one point of view, a happy ending.

LeQueux would remonstrate that this was not good, that the reader wanted to have the mystery solved and the guilty man punished. The doctor's answer to that was that the chief entertainment to be derived from one of his plots would be to show how easy it was for a man who really knew poisons to get away with murder. LeQueux still said no.

One night in January of 1910, when his affair with Ethel LeNeve was in its second year and still undiscovered, Crippen put in a rare appearance at one of his wife's social gatherings. Lil Hawthorne, Cora Crippen's variety-performer friend, was present. During the course of the evening, the Crippens and Lil Hawthorne got off to one side. Cora Crippen had some news for Miss Hawthorne which she wished to impart in the presence of her husband. 'Harvey and I,' she said, 'have decided to start life all over again. We've both done things that we're sorry for, but that's all in the past, isn't it, dear?' Crippen blinked happily and patted his wife's plump hand.

A few mornings afterward, Crippen walked into his office at Albion House and began to dictate a letter to Ethel LeNeve. The letter was to the Music Hall Ladies' Guild, and it was Cora Crippen's—rather, Bell Elmore's—letter of resignation as treasurer. The treasurer gave as her reason for resigning the fact that she had been called suddenly to the United States by the serious illness of a near relative. When Miss LeNeve had typed off the letter, Crippen signed it, 'Belle Elmore, per H.H.C.' Miss LeNeve remarked that it was odd that Mrs Crippen had not written the letter herself. 'She was too busy trying to get off to America,' said Crippen.

Lil Hawthorne was away in the Provinces on a variety tour when Mrs Crippen's resignation went in to the Guild. When she returned and heard about it, she sought out the doctor. 'This must of been very sudden,' Miss Hawthorne said, 'Cora leaving for America.' Crippen said it had been sudden. Miss Hawthorne asked who the near relative was who was so ill. 'It's a relative of mine, not Cora's,' said the doctor. 'He lives in San Francisco. There will be quite a bit of money involved, and one of us had to be there to protect our interests. I couldn't go, so Cora went.'

In the middle of March, some six weeks after Cora Crippen had gone away, Crippen sent a telegram to Lil Hawthorne. Cora was, the telegram stated, seriously ill in California. She had, it seemed, contracted pneumonia 'in the high mountains.' Miss Hawthorne called at Hilldrop Crescent and found Crippen practically off his rocker from worry. 'What would I do without Cora,' he wailed, 'now that we have started our new life together?' He seemed to become quickly rational at the sound of his own question. 'I would have to leave this house,' he said, '*that's* what I would have to do. It would be too full of memories.'

A few days later Lil Hawthorne got another telegram from Crippen. The worst had happened; Cora Crippen had passed on in California. The actress called on the bereaved husband. The associates of the deceased ex-treasurer of the Music Hall Ladies' Guild wished to pay their final respects; they wished to send flowers to the funeral. Where in California would the services be held? 'Cora wished to be cremated,' said Crippen. 'Her ashes will be returned here to me.'

Crippen inserted a paid notice of his wife's passing in a newspaper and went about his business. Lil Hawthorne called at his office a week later. The doctor was absent; so was Miss LeNeve. The actress learned from an employee of Albion House that Crippen had said something about a holiday in Dieppe, for a change of air to assuage his grief. Miss Hawthorne presumed that Crippen had given his secretary time off during his absence.

Upon his return from his holiday, greatly invigorated, Crippen appeared at a charity ball given by the Music Hall Ladies' Guild. He took Miss LeNeve. 'Cora bought two tickets before she left,' he explained, blinking at the ticket taker. 'No use wasting them, eh?'

Cora Crippen's theatrical acquaintances seemed set on making a production of the arrival of her ashes from America. Lil Hawthorne kept asking Crippen if the ashes had arrived yet. 'The ashes?' Crippen would repeat absent-mindedly. 'Oh, the *ashes*. No, they are not here yet.'

Late in June—more than four months after Cora Crippen had left on her fatal journey—an English variety actor named Nash, who had as many show-business acquaintances in New York as he had in London, returned from an American tour, including a series of engagements in and around New York. Nash had known Mrs Crippen, as Belle Elmore, and the two had many mutual friends in New York theatrical circles. Nash was startled to learn, upon returning to London, that Belle Elmore had died in the U.S.A. As he fell to thinking about the woman, it occurred to him that it was strange that none of her New York friends had heard of her death. He thought it stranger still that she had not communicated with a single one of her friends upon her arrival in New York en route to California.

Lil Hawthorne agreed with Nash. Now that Miss Hawthorne thought things over, she thought it was strange that Cora Crippen, her very dear friend, had not given her so much as the scratch of a pen after departing for the United States. Come to think of it, the whole business was queer—damned queer. Crippen had not mentioned a single detail relating to his wife's departure from London or her subsequent illness and death—what liner she had taken to America, whether she had died in a hospital or a private home, nothing.

Miss Hawthorne recalled that Crippen had brought his secretary, Miss LeNeve, to the charity ball of the Music Hall Ladies' Guild. That, now that she thought of it in a new light, had been an unusual thing to do on two counts. Crippen had certainly not been weighted down by grief over his wife's death, and he must have had some sort of social as well as business relationship with his secretary. Miss Hawthorne determined to find out just how well developed that social relationship was.

The actress called at Crippen's office in Albion House. The door was locked and her knocking went unanswered. Lil Hawthorne was sure she could hear whispers within. She knocked and she knocked and she practically busted the door down. Finally, Crippen answered. The actress looked past Crippen to his secretary. Miss LeNeve looked flushed. Miss LeNeve was, moreover, wearing a brooch and a necklace that Miss Hawthorne recognized as the property of her departed friend.

Lil Hawthorne was a lady who got around; she had connections. She was an acquaintance of Superintendent Frank Froest of Scotland Yard. She called on Superintendent Froest, laid the scanty facts relating to Cora Crippen's disappearance before him, and demanded action. 'What *kind* of action, Miss Hawthorne?' asked Superintendent Froest. '*Any* kind of action,' said the actress. 'Don't you think it's suspicious that that secretary of his is wearing his wife's jewelry and that his wife's ashes have never shown up?'

The Yard sprang into action; exactly eight days after Lil Hawthorne's call on Superintendent Froest, Inspector Walter Dew, a casually-gaited big gent with wing collar, a bowler and a cold-roast face, burst in on Dr Crippen at Albion House and suggested a spot of lunch. During a pleasant and unhurried repast, Inspector Dew cleared his throat, as if embarrassed by what he was about to say, and hinted to Crippen that there had been a bit of a complaint over at the Yard about Dr Crippen's secretary, a Miss LeNeve, having been seen wearing a necklace or some such thing that was the property of Mrs Crippen. 'I thought,' said Inspector Dew, 'that you could explain it, you know.'

Dr Crippen could indeed explain the jewelry. His wife had left London so hurried that she had neglected to take all of her belongings with her. And precisely what, asked Dew, had ever become of Mrs

Crippen anyway? Crippen let the Inspector in on a little secret. Mrs Crippen wasn't dead at all; she had run off with a man—a man with whom she had been carrying on for months. 'I thought enough of Cora,' Crippen explained, 'to hide what she had done. That's why I invented the story she had died.' Crippen blinked at the Inspector. 'And of course,' he continued, 'the whole business would have been very embarrassing for me, too.'

'To be sure, Doctor,' said Inspector Dew. 'To be sure. Tell me, who was the man?' A man named Bruce Miller—an actor, of all things. Inspector Dew stroked his handsome pepper-and-salt moustache. Bruce Miller. Bruce Miller. Why, of course. He had seen Bruce Miller in the music halls. A singer and dancer and story teller. 'A handsome chap, too, I *must* say,' said Inspector Dew. '*Too handsome*,' said Dr Crippen dryly. 'He is everything that I am not.'

'That young lady back in your office, Doctor,' said Dew. 'She's rather pretty, what?' Crippen confessed that he had taken up with Miss LeNeve after his wife had deserted him. Dew was thoughtful; he said he could understand a situation like that. 'Not to be condoned, you know,' was the way he put it, 'but completely understandable, old boy.'

Now that the whole thing had been cleared up, Dew said he must be getting back to the Yard. 'You know,' he confided, 'the person who complained against you tried to convince the Superintendent that your wife had met with foul play.'

'You don't have to tell me who *that* was,' said Crippen. 'I know. It was Lil Hawthorne.'

'How did you guess?'

'She's never had any use for me.' Dew was taking his leave when a thought came to Dr Crippen. 'I wish you would come out to the house and look around,' he said. 'Foul play is a pretty serious charge to make against a man.'

'Oh,' said Dew, 'that's quite unness'ry, old boy; it's perfectly *obvious* what happened. Perfectly.' But Crippen insisted. Dew reluctantly went to Hilldrop Crescent. He went through the house from attic to cellar. He was in the cellar with Crippen, consulting his watch and saying that he simply *must* be getting back to the Yard when Crippen pointed to the coal bin. 'You should really look at the brick floor under the coal,' said the Doctor. 'That would be the ideal place to hide a body in *this* house.' Dew looked pained, let out a little laugh with a hole in it, and strode over to the coal bin. The bin was practically empty and the brick floor was almost entirely visible. Dew poked at the floor with his cane. 'No body there,' he said, and hurried up the stairs and out of the house.

All this transpired, according to Dew himself, on Friday, July 8, 1910. On the following Monday afternoon, July 11, Lil Hawthorne called at the Yard. She wanted to know of Superintendent Froest what had happened in the Crippen matter. 'Nothing,' said Froest. 'The man's wife left him, that's all. That sort of thing is none of our concern, you know, Miss Hawthorne.'

Would it be any of the Yard's concern, the actress wanted to know, that Dr Crippen and Ethel LeNeve had disappeared over the week-end? Superintendent Froest summoned Inspector Dew and Dew strode over to Albion House. Sure enough, Crippen had gone, and the condition of his office indicated that he wouldn't be back, either. Miss LeNeve, too, had departed her lodgings.

A dental mechanic employed in Albion House told Inspector Dew that Dr Crippen had, the previous Saturday—the day after Dew had talked with Crippen—sent him out to purchase clothing for a boy of sixteen. The mechanic had purchased a brown tweed suit, stockings and boots, hat and overcoat.

Next day—Tuesday—Dew arrived at the conclusion that the clothing the dental mechanic had purchased for Crippen could have been for Ethel LeNeve to use as a disguise in a flight to somewhere with Crippen. The more Dew thought things over, the more suspicious he became. The records in the case from that point on are bleakly incredible. Dew went out to Hilldrop Crescent on the Tuesday to have another go at Crippen's house. While in the cellar, he remembered the little doctor's remark about the coal bin, poked at the brick floor, found nothing, and went back to the Yard again.

On the Wednesday, Dew was simply unable to shake off the feeling that something was amiss. He went out to the Crippen house a third time, and went down the cellar and poked at the floor of the coal bin for the third time in six days. He knocked around the rest of the house and, for the third time, left the Hilldrop Crescent trap without having come up with a thing.

Dew thought that it would perhaps be a good idea to backtrack on Dr Crippen's professional activities. He learned that the previous January, shortly before Cora Crippen had dropped from sight, Crippen had, in the name of Munyon's Remedies, gone to the drug house of Lewis and Burrows in New Oxford Street and asked for five grains of a powerful drug called hyoscin hydrobromide, which came in the form of small, soluble crystals. Lewis and Burrows had not had five grains of the drug on hand but had obtained it for Crippen from their wholesalers, the British Drug House. Crippen had put down, as the use for which he wished the drug, 'homeopathic preparation.'

The Munyon people had no record of the Crippen purchase having been used in any of their remedies. They suggested to Dew that Crippen had perhaps wanted the drug for his personal use. Dew consulted a couple of experts on drugs—Dr H.H. Willcox, senior analyst at the Home Office, and Dr Bernard Spilsbury, pathologist at St Mary's Hospital, and a noted witness for the Crown in many celebrated murder trials. Neither Dr Willcox nor Dr Spilsbury had ever heard of hyoscin hydrobromide being used in medicine. The stuff was used in injections but was certain death if taken orally.

On Wednesday—five days after his talk with Dr Crippen—Inspector Dew went out to Hilldrop Crescent and had his fourth shot at the coal bin. This time, for a totally inexplicable reason, he noticed something that had escaped him before: there was no mortar between some of the bricks. Removing the bricks was child's play. Guess what Dew found under the loose bricks—except the head.

Surgery and other marks on what was found identified the remains as those of Cora Crippen. Chemical analysis of the vital organs disclosed that the woman had been done in by a hearty draft of hyoscin hydrobromide.

The Yard printed up fliers describing Crippen and Miss LeNeve.

The author, LeQueux, recognized Crippen as the Doctor Adams who had tried to sell him a poison plot. The way LeQueux figured it, and the Yard too, was that Crippen, in superimposing his plot on actuality, had gotten rid of an unpleasant woman who stood in the way of a new love affair, and reduced expenses at the same time. But certainly Crippen had, on several counts, been stupid—as stupid, in fact, as Inspector Dew.

Late in July, a fortnight after Crippen and the girl had vanished, the Yard got a wireless from the captain of the S.S. Montrose, two days out of Antwerp for Quebec. He believed he had Dr Crippen and Miss LeNeve aboard as George Robinson, Sr. and George Robinson, Jr. He had become suspicious when he happened upon Robinson senior squeezing the hand of Robinson junior.

The Montrose was a nine-day tub. Inspector Dew caught the

Laurentic, which, weighing anchor from Liverpool, would just beat the Montrose to Quebec.

Dew intercepted Crippen and his paramour at Quebec and returned them to England. There the little doctor tried on a gallows for size. Ethel LeNeve, who obviously had not had any guilty knowledge of the murder, was, nonetheless, tried as an accessory after the fact. Upon being acquitted she vanished to wherever it is that victims in public scandals go. Before she disappeared, she remembered one thing. On the holiday to Dieppe, right after Mrs Crippen had lost her head, the doctor had carried a hatbox—one of those English leather hatboxes that the homicidal bellhop lugged around in *Night Must Fall*. During the Channel crossing the hatbox went missing. If what was in that hatbox could have talked it would probably have had something to say about people not being satisfied with the names they were born with.

BERNARD O'DONNELL
Angel-Makers of Nagzrev

This is not the story of one bad woman, but rather the story of a number of bad women—some fifty in all—who were responsible for a carnage of mass killing in which husbands, lovers, children and relatives were done to death without scruple or mercy. It was a *community* of murderesses who flourished in the remote Hungarian villages of Nagzrev and Tiszakurt and who rained death over the Valley of the Theiss. Fully to appreciate the nature of their murderous exploits it will be as well to get a bird's eye view of the setting for what can only be described as the most amazing poisoning drama the world has ever known.

Nagzrev is a settlement, five centuries old, situated on the largest tributary of the Danube, against a background of the broad rolling plains of Hungary, a smiling land of pastures and peasants where little has changed since it became the first home of the Asiatic Huns and the cradle of modern Europe.

Imagine the lonely little homesteads set amidst the wild vast plains, separated by miles of cornfields, self-contained, and self-ruled, with men and women living and dying in the shadow of their own homes. I do not know what the place is like now, but in 1929 there was not even a church within miles of the twin villages of Nagzrev and Tiszakurt. They had no doctor, no hospital, not even a trained nurse, only a few ancient crones who practised unhygienic midwifery and home cures and were called the 'wise women.' But their wisdom consisted only in preying on the ignorant folk who came to consult them. They were regarded with superstitious awe, and they played up to the beliefs which they had encouraged. Their homes were at once the village club, and the chemists shops where the sick bought drugs. They were also the beauty parlours where a love-sick girl could buy a 'potion' to win her lover. The 'wise women' combined the offices of nurse, confidante, and gossip-in-chief, called in at every birth, and summoned to perform the last rites in death, these dispensers of primitive medicines and wierd love-potions were the modern equivalent of the Zulu witch doctor.

Farming was the main industry of these two villages, but the 1914–18 war devastated large areas of Hungary and after the conflict there had not been enough to go round. Land was precious, so precious indeed that the aged owners grimly held on to their acres and only death would bring about a change of ownership. The centuries old law of single inheritance rendered more than one child, superfluous, since it meant another mouth to feed and here the 'midwife' had a useful role to play. These harpies had literally the power of life and death in the little communities they served, for the demise of children and even of elders and husbands, meant more land for the women who were left behind.

Thus, in return for some paltry gift—for the midwives were by no means gold-diggers in the modern sense of the word—the wise women would readily smother an unwanted child at birth, supply a 'charm powder' for the removal of a husband who had served his purpose or provide the means for any other 'removal job' that might be required. The ease with which the dispatch of the unwanted could be encompassed, gradually bred in the community a callous indifference to murder, while the lust for land became stronger than family ties. The axiom that blood is thicker than water did not mean much in the Theiss Valley, where murder and immorality stalked side by side from the year 1911, the year the first murder was discovered, until 1927 when the last crime was committed. Women indulged in an orgy of free love, interchanging their paramours without shame or compunction.

The village graveyards were full of men, women and children who had been murdered by arsenical poisoning obtained by steeping flypapers in water. How long these internicine murders might have gone on is beyond conjecture, for it was not until a young medical student decided to analyse the organs of a body washed up on the banks of the Tisza, that suspicions were aroused in the minds of the authorities. That chance analysis revealed the presence of an inordinate amount of arsenic in the body, and the police at once started enquiries as a result of which the bodies of Josef Nadarasz and Michæk Szabo were exhumed. It was found that they too had died from large doses of arsenic.

Suspicion fell on two midwives of the district, Susanna Olah (known as 'the White Witch of Nagzrev') and Frau Julius Fazekas. Anonymous letters to the police accused another midwife, Papy, of distributing arsenic to her customers. It soon became apparent to the authorities that they had uncovered a murder racket the like of which only a fiction writer could think up. The first woman pulled in by the police set the trial blazing. She confessed to a string of killings, the poison for which had been obligingly supplied by Frau Fazekas. The latter was obviously public enemy No. 1, so the police played a hunch on Frau Fazekas that paid off handsomely. They picked her up and after a thorough grilling, during which she denied everything, they let her go and, as the police anticipated she promptly went to the homes of all her 'customers' warning them that the game was up and terrifying them with dire threats if they dared to betray her. Hard on the heels of Frau Fazekas making her frantic calls were the detectives and thus in one grand round-up they were able to pull in every woman who had 'done business' with the purveyor of poison. All unsuspecting, Frau Fazekas returned to her home but two days later when the police arrived to take her in she lifted the poisoned chalice to her own lips and joined the host of fellow-villagers whom she had sped to the better land. A search of the evil-smelling den in which she had lived disclosed a vast pile of fly-papers ready for the sinister brew which had been Frau Fazekas' *specialité de la maison*.

Cheated of the arch-villainess of this appalling drama the police then went after another leading character, 'Susie' Olah. She was something out of Shakespeare's famous tableau, for 'Susie' was a frightening figure with piercing black eyes that glowed ruby-red at night. She lived in a hut with a fearsome collection of snakes and lizards which she trained to creep into the beds of her intended victims. To such a pitch can guilt and superstition bring human beings that some who were visited by these noisome reptiles believed they were bewitched and went mad.

The police found Susie Olah with her seventy-year-old sister Rosa Sebestyen, an old hag who acted as a go-between in negotiations with the former's clients. It was Rosa who passed on to Lydia Holyba, the arsenic with which she poisoned her ill-tempered ailing husband. This was a typical murder.

Husband Holyba was a sour-natured, dyspeptic man, who lay abed when he should have been working in the fields. A piece of land had to be sold to pay his debts, and this was considered the worst crime of which a husband could be capable. A desire for vengeance began to smoulder in Lydia Holyba's breast and when a handsome young labourer started to pay her court, her resentment against her useless husband flamed up.

For forty Hungarian pence she brought a packet of arsenic from Frau Sebestyen which she gave to her husband in a cup of coffee. He died in dire agony as do all victims of arsenical poisoning.

A particularly vile creature in this rustic horror was Juliana Lipka who confessed to no fewer than seven murders. In 1912 she poisoned her aunt whose savings, cottage and plot of land came to her through inheritance; nine years later her uncle followed the aunt to his grave and Juliana duly inherited his property too. Her stepmother, brother and sister-in-law were the next to be hurried out of the world, and their property also became hers. She finally achieved complete control of the family lands by the despatch of her own husband and another male relation. This harridan had hopes of marrying a young fellow of twenty-four despite her age and the fact that she was black-browed, pock-marked, squat and shapeless, with a most evil expression.

Another of the village women who admitted buying a 'potion' from the midwife Olah, was more resourceful in her defence. She declared that she genuinely believed that the 'medicine' she obtained would cure her husband of his drinking habits, which of course it did. He died within a few hours of taking the stuff.

More exhumations were made and more arrests followed, but the work of the police was hampered by the fact that gravestones had been swopped over, either by the prisoners before their arrest or by their accomplices, to the graves of persons who had died natural deaths. Many of the corpses unearthed contained enough arsenic to poison twenty men, and eventually over fifty women, young and old, were arrested in connection with the crimes.

Some of the stories told by the women when they reported the deaths of their husbands lacked nothing in subtlety or ingenuity. One declared: 'My man was never the same when he came back from the war. He had trouble which got worse and worse until he died.' And the quaint old village 'coroner,' as ignorant of the first principles of law as he was of medicine, would fumble for his pen and scrawl out a certificate of death.

The whole dread story of the family murders was unfolded at the trials of the fifty women who were described as 'The Angel-Makers of Nagzrev.' The proceedings held at the Szolnok Assize court, were spread over several months, and eventually some of the prisoners were sentenced to death and others sent to prison for life. There was only one prisoner who evoked some degree of sympathy, Elizabeth Molnar the twenty-year-old widow of Franz Molnar whom she was charged with murdering. It may provide a little light relief if I tell more fully how Elizabeth came to find herself in the dock, for she was vastly different from the other women on trial.

Elizabeth Molner possessed a slimness and grace which not even the thick, heavy garb of the peasant could hide, and her pale face with its frame of raven ringlets and crowned with the traditional head-dress presented a picture of haunting sadness. It was not a pose. Elizabeth was a native of the village of Tiszakurt, and at 17 she was the beauty of the place. She was carried off her feet by the tempestuous wooing of a youth named Molnar, the son of a small but quite well-to-do landowner in the neighbouring village of Nagzrev. He was a handsome young fellow this Molnar, and at the village dance that had followed the gathering of the harvest he cut a dashing figure, in his quaint traditional costume, which Elizabeth found irresistible. At first the marriage was happy enough, but before many months had passed shadows began to cloud the lustrous eyes of the girl-wife. Franz noted it but to his oft-repeated questions the girl assured him that nothing was worrying her.

But there was! A young villager of Tiszakurt with whom she had been more than friendly when Franz first appeared on the scene, had resented the abrupt termination of his association with Elizabeth. The disappointed suitor, Palinkas by name, quickly made it clear that he had no intention of being summarily dismissed. He crept up to the house one day while Franz and others of the household were busy in the fields and bluntly demanded that Elizabeth should still remain his sweetheart. He threatened to reveal certain imaginary secrets of their youthful flirtation and to bolster up the story he produced some indiscreet little notes that had passed between them. The girl knew she had nothing really serious on her conscience but she knew also that her husband was insanely jealous. But thereafter, when Molnar was away at neighbouring towns on business bent, there was a secret visitor at the Nagzrev farmhouse. It was this and the ever-present terror of discovery that brought shadows to displace the happiness in Elizabeth's eyes.

The time came when the distracted Elizabeth pondered the strange tales she had heard about Frau Fazekas, who, it was whispered possessed wierd charms and powers enabling wives to escape the thraldom of unwanted husbands or lovers. So one night, closely muffled up, Elizabeth slipped away from her home, and a little later tapped half-fearfully on the door of the midwife Fazekas' house. She pleaded for a charm—a magic something that would drive away the unwelcome youth Palinas and ensure her husband's continued love and his freedom from suspicion. That was how she explained her mission to Fazekas, whom she found sitting surrounded by bottles containing queer potions, and 'magic' cakes and confections. The midwife took up a small wheaten cake and pressed it into the visitor's hand. This cake, she said, was to be eaten only by the youth Palinkas, none other was to taste a single crumb, and from that moment Elizabeth could rest assured, Palinkas would cease to trouble her.

Clasping the small cake with its magic properties, Elizabeth sped back to her farmhouse, and a day or two later she found the opportunity she sought. Her husband announced he had to go into Szolnok to buy farming implements and would be away some time. As soon as he had departed Elizabeth, casting discretion to the winds in her eagerness to follow the witch's instruction, sent a message to Palinkas inviting him to have tea with her the following day. He duly arrived and amongst the things he ate at tea was the 'magic' cake. Though neither Elizabeth nor Palinkas knew it, the cake which Fazekas had prepared contained a lethal dose of arsenic and the witch's promise that never more would Elizabeth be troubled by her lover was horribly accurate. Within twenty-four hours he was dead.

Elizabeth was appalled by the dreadful manner in which the 'magic' cake has solved her problem, and gradually it dawned on her why Fazekas had become known locally as the 'windowmaker.' The death of her unrequitted lover now preyed on her mind and under the burden of her guilt she became morose and neurotic. One day when her husband teased her with a tit-bit of gossip to the effect that young Palinkas had died with her name on his pain-twisted lips, she flew into such a violent rage that her husband was at a loss to understand the reason for her outburst. But he began to lose a little interest in his sullen and unpredictable wife and his journeys away from home now became more frequent and of longer duration. This was enough to arouse suspicious in the distorted mind of Elizabeth and it soon became an obsession with her that Franz had found himself a lover.

She resolved that if she had lost the affections of her husband no one else should have them. There was a remedy. So to the evil Fazekas she went once more, this time with the full knowledge that the 'magic' she sought was the same deadly poison that had eliminated the ill-fated

Palinkas. Fazekas was ready to oblige and it remains to be recorded that within a matter of a few days a dry-eyed, half-crazed Elizabeth stood at the graveside of her husband, the handsome young Franz Molner.

Maybe it was because Elizabeth did not try to make excuses for herself or place the blame on the dead Fazekas, or perhaps it was her youthful beauty which softened the hearts of her judges. Anyway 'The Belle of Widow-Makers,' as the papers described her, escaped the death sentence and she was committed to penal servitude for life. While in gaol she attempted suicide declaring, 'I long only for death in which I shall again be united with the man I love.' Unfortunately there was no 'midwife' available to provide the 'magic' potion that could bring about this celestial reunion.

HAROLD EATON

The Benevolent Monster: Doctor Pritchard

Different types of murder merit different degrees of blame. If the swift blow, following upon strong provocation, be the most venial because it is the least premeditated, then murder by poison, being long prepared, is the most infamous. But even among poisoners there must be precedence; and the man who kills by administering a single fatal dose may well object to being ranked with the man who destroys his victim by slow torture. To the former class belongs Crippen; to the latter, Seddon, though probably more through inexperience than by design. Slow poisoning is the most subtle, perhaps the most artistic, method of murder, and upon the Continent there have always been many brilliant masters of this craft; but the acknowledged leader—one might almost say, founder—of the British School is Dr Edward William Pritchard.

Pritchard also has other claims to immortality. He committed his long-drawn-out crime for no discoverable reason—even the prosecution at the trial could not allege an adequate motive—and this fact alone renders his case unique. Moreover, he was the last convict to be publicly executed at Glasgow.

Though his trial took place in Scotland, England must bear the responsibility of his birth. His parents seem to have been people of some social standing, and he received a sound education. In 1846 he graduated at the Royal College of Surgeons, and later he travelled extensively in the Pacific, in Egypt, and in the Northern Polar Seas. During an interval between those voyages he set up in practice at Filey, in Yorkshire, where he married Mary Jane Taylor, daughter of Michael Taylor, a retired silk and lace merchant, who resided at the Grange, near Edinburgh. By her he had five children, of whom the eldest was thirteen at the time of the trial.

Ultimately, in 1859, as a result of this connection, he moved to Glasgow, where he succeeded in getting together a respectable practice, though it would appear that his financial position was never very sound and that he was usually in debt. Through his contributions to the papers upon such topics as cancer, gout, and the influence of vegetable medicines upon diseases, he achieved the reputation of a man of culture, a reputation that was enhanced by the active part which he played in the social life of the city. He was a prominent Mason, a director of the Glasgow Athenæum, and he won a considerable local fame by lecturing upon his voyages. It would appear, however, that his tongue travelled even farther than the rest of his body had done, for his descriptions of the Fiji Islands, to take one example, were never twice the same and possessed only one common feature, namely, a total lack of resemblance to the original. One gem from these lectures has been preserved and must be quoted because it illustrates the boastful figurative style of speech affected by the doctor: 'I have plucked the eaglets from their eyries in the deserts of Arabia and hunted the Nubian lion in the prairies of North America.' It must have been a remarkable spectacle.

Another illuminating story of Pritchard also deserves to be recorded. At one time he professed for Garibaldi, then at the height of his power, a prodigious admiration, which, without the doctor leaving Glasgow, ripened in the course of a week or so into a warm personal friendship. In order to quicken his regard for his hero, he presented himself with a walking-stick engraved with the following legend:

'To William Edward Pritchard from his friend General Garibaldi.'

Subsequently he elaborated this idea and tried to restore his warning professional reputation by writing himself testimonials from eminent London doctors.

Indeed, Pritchard's chief aim in life was to be thought well of by his fellows—a harmless enough vanity, had there been about him anything worthy to support it; but, as has been shown, the means which he employed to achieve this end were as ludicrous as they were inadequate. He flattered and bragged and lied to every one with whom he came into contact, and he even caused his photograph to be sold at considerably less than cost price by all the stationers in Glasgow in order that the humblest might be enabled to secure a memento of the eminent doctor, explorer, and friend of Garibaldi.

These efforts to win popularity do not seem to have met with much success. His professional brethren in the city took an immediate dislike to him, and others, though at a first meeting they were sometimes impressed by his effusive manner, generally discovered after a second interview the shallow pretentiousness of the man.

Photographs of Pritchard (zealously circulated by himself) show him to have been rather a dignified-looking person—what he would himself have described as 'a fine figure of a man.' His features were clean-cut, his eyes intelligent, and he wore an enormous but carefully-trimmed beard. Tall and portly, he had a commanding presence, and this allied to an almost embarrassing geniality gave the impression of adlermanic benevolence. Those who knew him best would have stigmatised him professionally as a charlatan, socially, as a hypocrite full of conceit and bombast. That he was a liar with an academic interest in forgery had already been suspected. His humbug he practised partly to further his popularity, but that he should commit without notice one of the most crafty and cruel murders of the century, would have been ridiculed by his bitterest enemy.

In 1863 any reputation that he had enjoyed was forfeited owing to a curious incident which was never properly solved. That it was capable of an innocent interpretation must be admitted, but the construction placed upon it illustrates the esteem in which Pritchard was held by his fellow-townsmen. The appropriate atmosphere is best introduced by a quotation from *The Glasgow Herald* of May 6th:

Lamentable Ocurrence
Young Woman Burned to Death

'Yesterday morning a melancholy incident occurred in the residence of Dr William Pritchard, situated at 11, Berkeley Terrace, Berkeley Street. The house, which is at the north side of the street, consists of two flats and attics, the servants' sleeping apartment being in the top flat fronting the street. About three o'clock one of the constables stationed in the vicinity of the dwelling observed the glare of fire through the attic window and immediately proceeded to the front door and rang the bell. The door was opened by Dr Pritchard, who slept in a bedroom on the second floor and who had been awakened a few minutes before the beell rang by his two sons, who slept in an adjoining apartment, calling out, "Papa." The doctor rose and, on opening the room door, was alarmed to find smoke in the lobby. . . . After leaving his boys in the lobby leading from the street door, he rushed up to the attic flat, pushed open the door of the servants' sleeping-room, and called out "Elizabeth," but received no reply.'

The report continued that ultimately, with the help of the constable, he forced his way into the room, where the body of one of the maids was discovered. The face, arms and trunk were badly charred, and only the legs encased in stockings had resisted the action of the flames. The obvious theory was that the girl, while reading in bed by candlelight, had fallen asleep and that the bedclothes had caught fire; stupefied by the smoke she must have been unable either to escape or to raise the alarm, and so had perished through a strange but not unprecedented mischance. An inquest was held, at which a verdict of Death by Misadventure was recorded, and there one might have thought the matter should have ended.

But this incident produced a crop of the most extravagant rumours. The fact that Miss Pritchard and the other servant were away upon that night was declared to be something more than mere coincidence. It was pointed out that no remains of any book had been found, and that the body, when discovered, was not contorted, but was lying peacefully, as though in slumber. These observations might perhaps be regarded as fair comment, but the scandal did not halt there. The most monstrous allegations, unsupported, as far as one can judge, by the slightest evidence, were made against the doctor. It was said that the girl was pregnant by her master and that the door of her room was locked upon the outside (an assertion, one would have said, most difficult of proof). Manifestly the implication was that Pritchard had either drugged or poisoned the girl and then completed or concealed his crime by setting fire to the house. The insurance company at first resisted his claim owing to these suspicious circumstances, but subsequently under threat of legal proceedings withdrew their objection, which could not possibly have been sustained by evidence.

It had always been the doctor's ambition to become the most talked about man in Glasgow, and he certainly succeeded in keeping his name in front of the public for close on two years; hardly had the scandal caused by this incident died down than a charge equally grave and more certain was launched against him.

It was in the autumn of 1864 that Pritchard began the systematic poisoning of his wife, with whom he had lived and apparently continued to live upon the most affectionate terms. That he was genuinely fond of his children there can be no doubt, and if he had ceased to care passionately for his wife, he could find, had, in fact, already found, consolation elsewhere without resorting to murder. The motive of his crime has baffled every psychologist who has attempted to review the case, and it would be impertinent after so long an interval to suggest causes which can now either be proved nor disproved.

It has been argued that he wished to get rid of her in order to marry his servant, Mary M'Cleod—he had, indeed, promised her that he would do so after his wife's death—but, as she had then been his mistress for several years, the urgency of this incentive is not apparent; and that she incited him to commit murder or that she was in any way accessory to the deed was expressly denied by Pritchard's confession. He would receive no pecuniary benefit from his wife's death, unless her mother had died in the meanwhile, and though he did indeed poison his mother-in-law a few weeks before he finally disposed of his wife, this second crime seems to have been purely subordinate and incidental to the first.

In fact, this total lack of motive would seem to suggest homicidal mania, yet such madness, one would think, must have betrayed itself in other ways; for it was not a sudden impulse, suddenly acted upon, but the slow torturing process of many months. Had the result in any way ministered to his love of admiration, one might have woven this murder into the general texture of the man's character, but if it remained undiscovered, it could only bring sympathy, tempered perhaps by suspicion. Either there must have been some secret motive which has escaped contemporary observers or this theory of homicidal mania must be upheld. If murder be one of the fine arts, then this indeed was art for art's sake.

At this Pritchard's household consisted of himself, his wife and five children, two servants, Mary M'Cleod and Mary Patterson, and two medical students who boarded with him in order to profit by his experience. If they contemplated studying toxicology, they could have found no abler master. The subtle blends of poisons that he used presents a fresh riddle. Did he think that a mixture of these preparations would render diagnosis more difficult and thereby lessen the chance of detection? Or was this the experimental zeal of the artist? Having found his subject he must not waste it upon one swift and certain process. The indictment charged him with poisoning his wife by the administration of tartarised antimony, aconitine and opium, or of one or more of them, and though the post-mortem examination only revealed the presence in considerable quantities of antimony, which, being a mineral poison, offered more resistance to the process of absorption, there can be little doubt that other preparations were also employed. According to his own account Pritchard never kept any drugs in the house save Battley's solution (opium) and chloroform—a strange lack of medicines for a doctor's house—but it was abundantly proved at the trial that his consulting-room was stocked not only with antimony, but with numerous other poisons, and that he had often purchased aconitine.

Up till October, then, Mrs Pritchard, never apparently a very strong woman, was enjoying normal health. Towards the end of that month, however, she became ill, and the symptoms of her malady, though not unusual, were severe. She began to lose strength and weight from frequent vomitings, and ultimately was forced to keep her bed for five days, owing to what she thought was a bad chill. Thinking that a change of air might do her good, she suggested to her husband that she should spend a few weeks with her parents at Edinburgh. To this request Pritchard immediately acceded, stipulating, however, that she should return to the bosom of the family for Christmas. How could the children enjoy their festivities without their mother? They must all try to prepare some little surprise to welcome her home again. Pritchard, it will be observed, was an excellent family man, and on Christmas evening could be relied upon, one feels sure, for an eloquent and affectionate speech, containing an entirely new anecdote about General Garibaldi. . . . Moreover, though his first experiment had been interesting, and though he was in no particular hurry, he did not wish to wait indefinitely.

Mrs Pitchard returned from her visit seemingly recovered; as she observed with some justification to her friends, she always enjoyed better health when she was away from home—a coincidence that could not be wholly attributed to the worries of housekeeping. Within a week of her homecoming the symptoms reappeared; frequent attacks of vomiting occurred, and on February 1st she suffered from a very severe attack of cramp.

Some few days after this, Dr Cowan, a relation of hers, visited her, and diagnosing her ailment as due to normal gastric trouble, prescribed small doses of champagne by way of stimulant. In spite of this the vomiting continued, and, as a natural result, her weakness increased. On February 8th she was seized with so violent an attack of cramp that she insisted upon Dr Gairdner being called in. To him Pritchard declared his opinion that his wife was suffering from gastric fever, but Dr Gairdner could find no symptoms indicative of this malady, and confessed that he was puzzled by the case.

Mrs Pritchard was now seriously ill, and on February 10th her mother came from Edinburgh to nurse her. Mrs Taylor was a hale old lady of seventy, and her only ailment seems to have been a frequently recurring attack of headache. For this she was in the habit of taking Battley's solution, which contains a fairly high percentage of opium, but she could not be regarded as a confirmed drug-taker; Pritchard's suggestion that she was addicted to drinking spirits is equally untrue.

On the 13th Mrs Taylor ordered for the patient some tapioca, which was left for some time on the table in the lobby. Subsequently a cupful of this was made and taken by Mary M'Cleod to the sick-room. Whether the invalid took any is not clear, but both Mrs Taylor and the cook tasted it and were immediately seized with violent retching. So severe was the attack that Mrs Taylor declared that she must have contracted her daughter's illness—a shrewder diagnosis than many a doctor could have made.

It is possible that she taxed Pritchard with having tampered with the food, though this does not seem likely, for she certainly communicated her suspicions to no one else; or perhaps Pritchard realised that if her death occurred before that of her daughter he would inherit a certain amount of money, or again he may have seen in her just another subject for his experiments. Whatever the reason, he decided that her death would be convenient, might even be necessary. It would isolate his victim; it would help him financially; it would test the truth of his theories. But there was nothing precipitate about Pritchard; he was, it would seem, a very conscientious and patient poisoner—no sudden *coup-de-théâtre*, but several restrained and carefully thought-out scenes working up to the climax.

It was not until February 24th that Pritchard decided to complete his less important murder. About nine p.m. the bell of Mrs Taylor's room pealed violently, and the servant, on answering it, found the old lady in a state of collapse. Hardly able to speak, she demanded hot water in order to induce vomiting, but this remedy proved unavailing, and she soon passed into a condition of coma. Pritchard, apparently much upset, sent one of the medical students to fetch the nearest doctor, and soon afterwards Dr Patterson, who lived within two hundred yards of the house, arrived. The scene which ensued is best described in his own words:—

'Dr Pritchard met me in his hall and conducted me to the bedroom, telling me that his mother-in-law, whilst in the act of writing a letter, had fallen off her chair on to the floor and been conveyed upstairs about half an hour before I came.' (This, of course, was pure invention.) 'She and his wife, said the prisoner, had partaken of some bitter beer for supper, and soon after, both became sick and vomited and complained of its being more bitter than usual. . . . I asked in regard to the previous state of his mother-in-law's health and particularly as to her social habits, when he led me distinctly to understand that she drank spirits occasionally. . . .

'On entering the bedroom I observed Mrs Taylor lying on the edge of the bed nearest to me on her right side, with all her clothes on. She had all the appearance of a sudden seizure. Mrs Pritchard, in her nightdress and nothing on her head, and her hair very much dishevelled, was in the same bed, but underneath the bedclothes, sitting up immediately beyond her mother. Mrs Taylor was then alive, and she gave me the impression of a healthy-looking old lady and previously in very good health . . . a very superior-looking person, not having the slightest appearance of being addicted to the use of spirituous or intoxicating liquors. Her face was rather pale, but the expression was calm and placid. The eyelids partially closed; the lips rather pale and livid; the breathing slow and laborious; the skin cool and covered with a clammy perspiration; the pulse imperceptible, and she seemed to me perfectly unconscious. On my opening up the eyelids I found both pupils very much contracted. From these symptoms and judging from her general appearance, my conviction was that she was under the influence of opium or some other powerful narcotic, and I at once pronounced my opinion that she was dying. . . . Pritchard said she had frequently had attacks of a similar kind before but never one so severe.

'The old lady lay apparently comatose or unconscious, but on being roused a little and the head and shoulders slightly elevated, a degree of consciousness returned and the pulse became susceptible at the wrist. . . . Pritchard clapped the old lady on the shoulder and said: "You are getting better, darling," I looked at him ominously, as much as to say, "Never in this world." . . . The coma returned and the breathing became more oppressed and more laboured. . . .

'I left the room and went downstairs with Pritchard to his consulting-room, and there repeated my opinion that she was in a state of narcotic-ism. Pritchard then said that the old lady was in the habit of regularly using Battley's sedative solution, and that she had a few days before purchased not less than a half-pound bottle of that medicine and that it was very likely that she might have taken a good swig at it. My impression was that she was not what is called an opium-eater.'

It may be noted that this bottle was discovered when the corpse was being dressed, and on being submitted to chemical analysis was found to be charged with antimony and aconite.

Dr Patterson went home at half-past eleven, and about one in the morning he was again summoned, but realising the hopelessness of the case, refused to go. A few days later Pritchard called upon him, and telling him that Mrs Taylor had died about an hour after his departure, asked him to make out the death certificate. This Patterson declined to do, and when the Registrar sent him the ordinary form to fill up, he returned it blank with the following comment:

'I am surprised that I am called to certify the cause of death in this case. I only saw the person for a very short period before her death. She seemed to be under some narcotic; but Dr Pritchard, who was present from the first moment of the illness until death occurred (and this happened in his own house) may certify the cause. The death was certainly sudden, unexpected, and to me, mysterious.'

Pritchard, therefore, was forced to make out the certificate himself. Apoplexy following upon paralysis was his verdict, but it may be pointed out that paralysis follows, not precedes, apoplexy; this inversion is typical of the doctor's medical knowledge, for as Dr Gairdner put it in the witness-box, 'he was not a model of wisdom, accuracy, and caution in applying names to things.' Why, with the whole dictionary of diseases to choose from, he should have selected these is hard to say, for Dr Patterson declared that no such symptoms existed; but it may be that Pritchard wished to substantiate his lie that Mrs Taylor was a drunkard and a drug-taker.

Having disposed of his first victim, without awakening suspicion in any one save Dr Patterson, Pritchard was now enabled to devote his whole attention to his wife. The shock of seeing her mother die, lying beside her in the same bed, had greatly weakened her, and but a little was needed to finish this second murder, yet Pritchard with a refinement of cruelty, seems to have abstained for several days from administering further doses of poison—presumably in order that a decent interval might separate the deaths of mother and daughter.

It is not the least curious feature of this case that Pritchard should have invited the one man who already suspected him to witness his second crime. Dr Patterson was manifestly hostile to him, and his conduct over Mrs Taylor's death certificate should have warned Pritchard that he was not an easy man to hoodwink. Palmer[1] chose octogenarians for his innocent accomplices, and had Pritchard observed similar precautions it is probable that his crimes might have escaped detection. Like Lamson's[2] voluntary return from France, it was a bold stroke, but it only served to furnish complete evidence of his guilt.

On March 1st Pritchard accidently met Patterson and asked him to come and see his wife, which he did the following day. He had, of course, seen her previously upon the night of Mrs Taylor's death, and his first impression of her—an impression which he gave in evidence at the trial—is, if really received at the alleged time, most remarkable.

'She seemed,' he said, 'exceedingly weak and exhausted. Her features were sharp, or thin, with a high hectic flush on her cheeks, and her voice was very weak and peculiar—in fact, very much resembling a person verging into the collapsed stage of cholera. . . . At first I was inclined to attribute her appearance to the recent severe attack of gastric fever which I was told by the prisoner she had had. . . . At the same time I must say that I could not banish from my mind the idea, or rather conviction, that her symptoms betokened that she was under the depressing influence of antimony—that conviction came upon me in her presence and I could not get quit of it. I did not put a single question to her.'

The prejudice, one may say the vindictiveness, of this evidence is apparent, and one questions whether, without any examination of the patient, such a strange theory ever entered his head. His description of this second visit lacks none of the animosity of his first impression.

'She was in bed, still very weak and prostrate, and in a weak voice expressed her satisfaction and her gratitude at my calling. Then in a very earnest manner, she asked me if I really thought that her mother was dying when I saw her. I said most decidedly I did, and had told Pritchard so. She then clasped her hands, looked up and feebly exclaimed, '*Good God, is it possible?*' and burst into a flood of tears. I put some questions then as to her mother's previous state of health, especially if she was habitually addicted to the use of Battley's solution. She told me that her mother's health, generally speaking, was good, but that she suffered occasionally from what she called neuralgic headaches, and for relief of these attacks she did take a little Battley's solution, but she added that she could not be said to be in the habitual use of that medicine.'

He prescribed various drugs and food for her, and on March 5th Pritchard called on him and reported that his wife was better for his advice, but still very weakly and her stomach irritable. Patterson's suspicions, formed on the night of February 24th and strengthened by this second visit, do not seem to have forced him to take any action.

He saw her for the third and last time on the evening of March 17th, when Pritchard came round himself and asked him to come and see her.

'I have always attended my wife in all her ailments of every kind during the whole period of our married lives, now fifteen years, and some of these illnesses were very severe; but I never saw her so ill as she was on the occasion which terminated fatally.'

This is a platitudinous beginning, but the doctor gradually warms to his theme.

'I gave my wife no medicines during her illness excepting wine, champagne, and brandy; I trusted to Nature to right itself with the assistance of these restoratives. During the last six weeks her power of sleeping entirely went away. . . . I then wrote to her mother to come and nurse her, and she arrived about February 11th; her arrival had a beneficial effect upon Mrs Pritchard for some time, but still the sleeplessness continued. . . .

'After her mother's death, she became rapidly worse; indeed I ascribed her decease to the agitation consequent upon her mother's death. At the time of the last event she was strongly impressed with the idea that she herself would die on a subsequent day at exactly the same hour. On the night preceding her death she was apprehensive that, unless she got sleep, she should not get through the night. I sent for Dr Patterson, who came immediately and afterwards dictated a prescription. . . .

'She got the first draught as prescribed by Dr Patterson about ten o'clock, but she said after drinking it that it was not half strong enough, and asked if she might have some of her mother's medicine (Battley's solution). I refused . . . she then asked me to come to bed, as I must be tired with the weary nights of watching. It was then about midnight. I tried to persuade her that I should sit up to watch her till past the time when her mother had died; but to please her I got into bed and almost immediately I fell asleep from the state of exhaustion I was in; I was awakened by her pulling at my beard, and found my wife struggling to get into bed. She appeared to have got out of bed. She said, "Edward, I am faint." I assisted her into bed and asked how long I had been asleep, but she answered, "Don't speak. Look! Do you see my mother?" I said, "No; it is only a vision; only imagination." She said she felt cold and I need try no more skill; that I had failed this time and that she was going to her mother. I got alarmed and rang the bell violently and the youngest servant came. I desired her to make a mustard plaster as quickly as she could, and on that my wife turned round and said, "Edward, I'm in my senses; mustard plasters will do no good," and almost immediately she fell back in my arms and died.'

Whether there is any truth in this story of her premonition or whether it was merely a theatrical invention of Pritchard's cannot, of course, be decided, but she did in fact draw her last breath at almost precisely the same minute at which her mother had died on February 24th.

After having been charged with also causing the death of Mrs Taylor, Pritchard voluntarily made the following statement in reference to this second accusation:—'I never administered poison to her. I did and do believe that she died from paralysis and apoplexy. I have no further statement to make, and by the advice of my agent will make none, with the exception that I am entirely innocent of the charge preferred against me.'

The trial opened at the High Court of Justiciary, Edinburgh, in July, 1865, before the Lord Justice Clerk (Right Hon. John Inglis), Lord Ardmillan and Lord Jerviswoode. The Solicitor-General (afterwards Lord Young), Mr Gifford and Mr Chrichton appeared for the prosecution, while counsel for the panel (i.e. prisoner) were Mr Rutherford Clarke, Mr Watson and Mr Brand.

Scottish practice does not admit of opening speeches in criminal causes, and the Court proceeded at once to the hearing of the evidence. Details of the illness of Mrs Pritchard were given by the various members of the doctor's household, but the most important witness for the Crown was naturally Dr Patterson. In his examination-in-chief, which has already been extensively quoted, he exhibited such an obvious bias against the prisoner that the defence were able to suggest with some success that his prejudice rendered his evidence untrustworthy. One may perhaps differentiate, as did the Lord Justice Clerk, between dislike of the prisoner as a man and dislike of the prisoner arising from a conviction of his guilt, but any display of feeling by a witness is highly undesirable.

Dr Patterson's evidence, moreover, is noteworthy for its strange conception of a doctor's duty; one hears nowadays much talk of allowing medical men to please 'professional privilege,' and to refuse to answer questions relating to a medical confidence; there is a great deal to be said for this doctrine, but Patterson's code of professional etiquette will find few supporters.

Having stated in answer to counsel for the Crown that as soon as he saw Mrs Pritchard he came to the conclusion that she was 'under the depressing influence of antimony,' the doctor was subjected to a brief but damaging cross-examination by Mr Rutherford Clarke.

'Did you mean to convey to us that she had been taking antimony medicinally or that she was being poisoned by antimony?'—'My impression that she was being poisoned by antimony.'

'As you thought that Mrs Pritchard was suffering in that way from antimomy, did you ever go back to see her again?'—'I did not, and I believe I never would have been called back again if I had not met Pritchard accidentally in the street.'

'Why did you not go back?'—'Because she was not my patient, I had nothing to do with her.'

'Then, though you saw a person suffering from what you believed to be poisoning by antimony, you did not think it worth your while to go near her again?'—'It was not my duty. I had no right to interfere in any family without being invited.'

'Dr Patterson, is it not your duty to look after a fellow creature who, you believe, is being poisoned by antimony?'—'There was another doctor in the house. I did the best I could by apprising the Registrar' (over Mrs Taylor's death certificate).

'Did you tell Dr Pritchard?'—'I did not. Had I been called into consultation with another medical man I should certainly have considered it my duty to have stated distinctly my medical opinion.'

'But you stood upon your dignity and did not go back to see what you believed to be a case of poisoning?'—'I had no right.'

'No right?'—'I had no power to do it.'

'No power?'—'I was under no obligation.'

'You were under no obligation to go back to see a person whom you believed was being poisoned with antimony?'—'I took what steps I could to prevent any further administration of antimony.'

'By never going back to see her?'—'No. By refusing to certify the death. Had there been a post-mortem examination of Mrs Taylor's body, I believe that in all probability the drugging with antimony would have gone no further—at least that time.'

'Having been in a house where you thought there was poisoning going on, you did not consider it your duty to go back?'—'I had discharged my duty so far as I thought it incumbent upon me.'

'By prescribing certain things and not knowing whether the prescription was followed?'—'In any case, where a consultation is held the consulting physician has no right to go back to see the patient.'

'Then it was the dignity of your profession that prevented you from going back?'—'It is the etiquette of our profession. That was one reason why I did not go back. I did not say it was the only one. In any case, when I had been called in for consultation, were I to go back it would be a breach of etiquette of my profession.'

The position adopted by Patterson became the subject of much controversy at the time, and he himself wrote several long letters to the papers in vindication of his attitude. But regarded from either stand-point, his conduct is equally unjustifiable. If he really came to the conclusion that Mrs Pritchard was being poisoned he could not shelter himself behind a professional scruple; one can imagine no rule more dangerous than that one class should arrogate to itself the right to decide, according to its private code of etiquette, whether it will assist or hamper justice. If, on the other hand, Dr Patterson's opinion was formed subsequently, comment upon his evidence is superfluous.

The expert witnesses called by the Crown were Drs Maclagan, Littlejohn and Penny; of these the first two had conducted the post-mortem examinations while Dr Penny had submitted portions of the remains to further chemical analysis. According to the excellent practice of the Scottish courts these witnesses gave formal certificates 'on soul and conscience,' and no personal examination was allowed until these declarations had been read in court.

In the case of Mrs Taylor, antimony was discovered in all the organs, but though the bottle of Battley's solution which, in the submission of the Crown, was supposed to have caused death, was found to be charged with aconitine, no trace of this latter poison was revealed. It shows the fairness and thoroughness with which these investigations were conducted that Dr Maclagan's certificate ends with the following paragraph:—

'As Mrs Taylor's body had been exhumed, I thought it my duty to examine some of the earth in which it had been interred, though this was superfluous from the fact of the soil being dry and the coffin entire; it was not found to contain a trace of soluble antimony, and was therefore incapable of impregnating with this metal any body buried in it.'

The post-mortem examination of Mrs Pritchard, though likewise showing the presence of antimony in considerable quantities, presented distinctive features. The stomach was entirely free from any trace of poison, while only a small deposit was found in the intestines. From this Dr Maclagan inferred that antimony had not been administered in any great quantity within a few hours of death. Owing to the fact that all the organs and fluids of the body were impregnated with the poison, he was of opinion that antimony must have been taken in repeated doses extending over some considerable period, though he could not by any chemical process determined the extent of that period.

Recalled after Dr Penny had given the result of some further experiments, Dr Maclagan declared that all the symptoms in Mrs Pitchard's case indicated poisoning by antimony, and that 'there was nothing in the case to suggest to a medical man of ordinary intelligence that she was suffering from gastric fever or any other fever.'

In order to prove that the prisoner had been in possession of these poisons, witnesses were called who deposed to the fact that Dr Pritchard had made large and frequent purchases both of antimony and aconitine, and must therefore have maintained a greater stock of these drugs than any other practitioner in the city. Almost the only evidence called by the defence was in rebuttal of this testimony, and though Mr Clarke established that other doctors were in the habit of buying large amounts of the same poisons, the fact remained that Pritchard had at least sufficient to have accounted for a dozen more victims.

In his able address to the jury the Solicitor-General laid down certain propositions. It was contestable that although none bf the medicines prescribed for the two ladies had contained antimony, antimony in large quantities had been found in their bodies. That this could have been taken accidentally was denied by the prisoner's own statement, and that any one should commit suicide by so painful and lingering a method was inconceivable. The prisoner had many opportunities of administering antimony, and he had antimony in his possession.

It was all very convincing save when counsel dealt with the question of motive. He sought to establish the fact that Pritchard would derive some small pecuniary benefit from the death of these two women, but it seems indisputable that the murder of Mrs Taylor was incidental to the murder of the prisoner's wife; that crime had been conceived and initiated long before the chance for this second murder arose. That murder had been committed was beyond doubt; who, then, was the murderer?

'The only two grown persons, except the boarders, who were in the house during that time,' declared the Solicior-General,' the only two who had access to the patients, were the prisoner at the bar and Mary M'Cleod. This is narrowing the case to a very short question. I have excluded every other idea from the case, by fair, legitimate, convincing argument, upon evidence that is not open to dispute. I have excluded the notion of natural death. I have established the fact of death by poison. I have excluded the idea of death by accident, by suicide, by administration medicinally. . . . I find that the only two who had access to these miserable victims and had any opportunity to perpetrate the murders were the prisoner and this one girl. Now pray consider with respect to the wife, upon the question whether or no the prisoner is not the man clearly proved by irresistible evidence to be so, what was the nature of the murder? It was a murder in which you almost detect a doctor's finger.'

For the defence, Mr Clarke naturally tried to escape through the loophole presented to him by the Solicitor General. The prosecution had shown that the murders must have been committed either by

Pritchard or by Mary M'Cleod, but had they demonstrated the guilt of one or the innocence of the other? Both had equal opportunities, but they had only heard the evidence against one. In effect the Crown asked them to choose between the prisoner at the bar and one of the witnesses.

A point which he might have emphasised and which he seems to have neglected, is the question of motive. M'Cleod must have had, in the death of Mrs Pritchard, far more interest than any alleged by the prosecution against the doctor himself; for, in the event of his wife's death, her master had promised to marry her—a marriage which, apart from any affection she may have felt for Pritchard, would give her, a servant-girl of seventeen, an assured position in the world.

As might have been expected, Mr Clarke had some strong things to say about Dr Patterson, and the way in which he had given his evidence; but though he could comment upon the manner, the matter remained. A Scottish jury is not so apt to be influenced by rhetoric as is an English one.

In an exhaustive and scrupulously fair summing-up the Lord Justice Clerk omitted no point which might tell in favour of the prisoner; but, though by Scots law a third verdict of 'Not Proven' may be returned, the jury, after an hour's deliberation, found the prisoner guilty on both counts.

Pritchard, it seems, had throughout been confident of acquittal, and upon hearing the verdict he almost collapsed. Recovering his composure almost at once he listened calmly to the judge's exhortation to make his peace with God. While the sentence was being passed he occasionally nodded as though in acquiescence and then, after bowing with something of his old dignified flourish to the court, he was led, still smiling and acknowledging his friends, to the prison-van.

It was not to be expected that any petition for mercy would be raised, but Pritchard at once tried to create a favourable atmosphere by confessing his guilt and naming Mary M'Cleod as the real instigator of the crime. Finding, however, that this story obtained no credence, he recanted, and admitted that he and he alone was responsible for the murder of both his wife and his mother-in-law.

In prison his conduct, if sincere, was exemplary. He spent most of his time in devotion and seemed to derive much comfort from the ministrations of the chaplain, but with so great a hypocrite it may be doubted whether this piety was anything more than a pose—a recrudescence of that old desire to be thought well of by his fellows.

One genuine and redeeming trait in his character must, however, be recorded, and that was his affection for his children; an affection which seems to have been returned, for his eldest daughter, aged thirteen, wrote a pathetic letter to the prison authorities begging them to be kind to 'dear papa.' One other letter, too, must be noted, for it is not the doctor's least astonishing achievement; it may be, though, that the wording rather than the sentiment makes it sound grotesque. Written on the eve of his execution, it is addressed to the son and the brother of the women he had murdered:

> 'Farewell, brother, I die in twenty hours from this—Romans viii. 34–39. Mary Jane, darling mother, and you I will meet, as you said the last time you spoke to me, under happier circumstances. Bless you and yours prays the dying penitent.
> 'EDWARD WILLIAM PRITCHARD.'

On July 29th the convict was executed with all the pomp and circumstance of medieval justice, and throughout the interrogations and processions he bore himself with dignity and courage. It may be said of him as of many another great criminal that he died better than he had lived.

The scene was enacted in Jail Square, close to Hutcheson Bridge, and was witnessed by a crowd of nearly 100,000 most of whom had assembled overnight. The modern 'drop' had not then been invented and the slow, primitive process contrasts with the swift method employed to-day. 'This scaffold,' says *The Edinburgh Evening Courant* of that date, 'is a large, black-painted box, the interior of which is about 12 feet square, the sides rising × feet above the platform. The height of the beam is about 8 or 9 feet, and the rope was placed so as to let the culprit fall between 3 and 4 feet. The frame of the scaffold is on wheels and is put together for the most part with bolts. The platform is reached by a broad flight of steps. Underneath the scaffold, as usual, a coffin was placed. It was a plain black shell and certainly appeared scarcely long enough for the body it was to contain.'

As the procession came into view of the crowd there was some jeering, but this soon died away and it was in complete silence that Callcroft the executioner, drew the bolt. Pritchard appeared to suffer great agony, for he was seen to shrug his shoulders about a dozen times, and only after Callcroft had gone beneath the scaffold and straightened the legs, did all movement cease.

Not much that is good can be said of him. He loved his children; he met his death with dignity; but he was a braggart, a hypocrite, and one of the most cruel murderers in the history of crime. To become popular had always been his ambition; he left behind him a record the infamy of which is not yet wholly forgotten.

JOHN LAWRENCE
An Indian Holocaust

Behind the veil of the East are hidden untold tragedies and horrors. The veil is seldom torn aside, but when it is there is revealed a scene which is only understandable but faintly to the Western mind. It is only occasionally that some crime is brought to light which contains all the elements of a similar tragedy of the West. Even then it usually reveals some bizarre element, something which lifts it out of the ordinary rut, and stamps it definitely as being of the East, despite the fundamental passions which underlie it.

In 1911 there were living in Meerut a Mr Fulham and his wife. Mr Fulham was an assistant examiner of military accounts. The two were friendly with a Lieutenant Clark and his wife who lived at Agra. Lieutenant Clark, a Eurasian officer in the Indian Subordinate Medical Service, frequently corresponded with Mrs Fulham and she with him. The two families were perhaps more intimate than most similar families would be in England, and that intimacy was to result in six deaths directly and at least one other indirectly.

Early in their acquaintanceship Lieutenant Clark and Mrs Fulham formed a *liaison*. Neither was young—both were in the middle forties—and there was no excuse that they were swept from their feet by the uncontrolled desires of youth. The two were certainly overwhelmed by one desire, and that was to be married. But the obstacles in their way were Mr Fulham and Mrs Clark.

It was decided to remove Mr Fulham first. With Clark living in Agra at the time and the Fulhams in Meerut, the task devolved on Mrs Fulham. Clark, by his position in the medical service, had a ready access to any drugs and poisons he wished, and he made full use of his knowledge. Regularly he wrote to Mrs Fulham, sending her drugs and

227

giving her instructions how they should be administered so that no suspicion should be aroused. And regularly she replied, reporting progress. No fewer than four hundred of her letters were found, and these letters of themselves tell a most remarkable story in the history of crime.

It was early in 1911 that Mr Fulham began to complain of not feeling well, of suffering from the heat and from stomach troubles. Hardly anything he ate agreed with him, and finally he became so ill that he was removed to hospital for treatment. There Major Palmer, of the Royal Army Medical Corps, diagnosed heat stroke. Mr Fulham was unconscious when he was brought in, his face was purplish, and he had frequent convulsions. But under the care of the hospital doctors Mr Fulham made a rapid recovery and was able to return home.

At home Mr Fulham did not remain for long. The alarming symptoms which had compelled his removal to hospital in the first place, returned with redoubled vigour. They were again diagnosed as being due to heat stroke. Mrs Fulham appeared to be very upset by her husband's illness and was a constant visitor at the hospital. The weather that year was unusually hot, and there had been an abnormal number of cases of heat stroke, so that the illness of the assistant examiner of military accounts did not excite any suspicion.

This time Mr Fulham did not make so rapid a recovery. When he left the hospital he was very weak. He had been under treatment for some time and when he left he decided to go to Agra to try to recuperate. He arrived there on October 8th, and on the 10th he was dead. Within twenty-four hours he was buried and one of the obstacles to the marriage of Lieutenant Clark and Mrs Fulham had been removed.

There was Mrs Clark. She, too, began to complain of feeling ill, but hers was a tougher constitution than Mr Fulham's. The months slipped by and the lovers became more and more impatient.

It was not until over a year after the death of the assistant examiner of military accounts that Mrs Clark died. On the afternoon of November 18th, 1912, Lieutenant Clark left his home and paid a visit to Mrs Fulham. Before he left he told his wife to be careful as there were thieves about.

Late that night Clark's daughter was wakened by her mother's screams for help. She rushed into her mother's bedroom and saw a native standing beside her bed with a heavy stick in his hand. Her mother was bleeding from a number of wounds and could barely speak.

Half an hour later Lieutenant Clark returned. He usually was home by ten o'clock, but it was significant that that night he did not return until one o'clock. Mrs Clark died without recovering consciousness and there immediately began a search for the native or natives who had attacked her.

Rumour had been busy with the names of Lieutenant Clark and Mrs Fulham, and when the police began to examine Clark's native servants suspicion was quickly aroused. A man named Budhu was arrested and he immediately broke down. As a result of the remarkable story he told, the police not only arrested Lieutenant Clark and Mrs Fulham but three natives. A search of Clark's bungalow brought to light first of all a diary which Mrs Clark kept and secondly a steel box in which there were some four hundred letters which had been writen to Clark by Mrs Fulham.

But first the story of the native servant Budhu.

'My master wanted me to put poison in the memsahib's food,' he related. 'He gave me a bottle of stuff to put in her tea and it made her very sick. Later he asked me if I could arrange to kill the memsahib, and I saw Sukhia (one of the accused natives) and offered him a hundred rupees. Sukhia replied, "I cannot do it for a hundred rupees. I want more." A week later I arranged to carry out the sahib's wishes for six sovereigns and ten rupees.

'About one o'clock four of us went to the memsahib's bungalow. I waited on the verandah while the others went in at the back door, but a dog barked. Just at that moment the memsahib's husband rode up on a bicycle and he locked the dog in an outhouse and stopped it barking. The memsahib was then killed. We heard someone cry out and we ran off.'

Both Mrs Fulham and Clark denied the story that was told.

'Bodhu has made it up because I was very strict with him,' he declared. 'I never instigated anyone to murder my wife. Thieves murdered her. The only thing missing from the house is money, which I gave her on November 16th. The whole case against me is false. I am innocent.'

But the letters of Mrs Fulham's, practically every one of which her lover had kept, were damning. They not only proved that the two had been plotting the death of Mrs Clark but what had not been previously suspected, that they had murdered Mr Fulham. The prosecution relied largely upon these letters to prove their case, and never had there been more damnatory documentary evidence available for such a purpose.

Clark had kept each letter in its original envelope, and had initialed each one as he had answered it. The letters in themselves form a unique history of the crime, and are among the most psychologically interesting letters ever published.

'In your presence,' wrote the infatuated woman to her lover, 'I seem to melt and become like wax instead of being strong and making you listen to me, sweetheart darling. My hubby is very angry. It appears he saw you talking to me at my bedroom door. He did not see anything beyond our whispering, but that was enough to make him jealous and angry. How hard it is to struggle against such odds and disadvantages. I can only ask you to wait for me till I come to you free and unfettered.'

On April 24th, 1911, she wrote:

'I have given the tonic regularly. It is a very good tonic. My hubby is quite well and strong. It really seems to have done him good.'

Two days later she was writing, 'Hubby seems quite unaffected by the tonic. In fact, he is stronger and better than before.'

A letter shortly afterwards contained the significant words, 'Oh! what a different wife your second one will be. The stakes are high, but the prize is well worth striving after.' This was followed by a letter in which she wrote, after reporting the failure of the latest powders to act, 'Do consider and hit on a plan which will soon achieve our most deserved and longed-for results.'

Step by step the progress of the conspiracy may be read in these terrible letters. On July 18th she was writing, 'Really, I don't know how he escapes getting heatstroke, as he is in a very favourable condition for it. His eyes are bloodshot, and his face is at times almost purple.'

Mrs Fulham later asserted that she was so much under the influence of her lover that she could not refuse to carry out his wishes. Her letters do not bear our this assertion. In different letters she wrote, 'You assure me you are determined to win me at any cost. Come what may I will help you to achieve that end. I don't approve of your powders at all. How many hundred years will it take?'

She wrote constantly asking his advice and full details of the symptoms she could expect so that she could see whether the drugs were acting or not. He was ill after a dinner and she commented, 'Hubby is very ill with symptoms of cholera. All blame the Masonic dinner, but you and I know. I cannot bear to see his suffering.'

She could not bear it because she wanted it over quickly. She did not hesitate to suggest to her lover that he might try some of his drugs on

Mrs Clark. 'Do you think the same symptoms could be produced on someone we know?' she wrote, and when Clark promptly fell in with her suggestion she replied, 'You must not attempt to free yourself so soon as next month, as it would look very bad in the eyes of the world. You have grown-up children, who might notice your anxiety to become a widower as soon as Mrs Fulham is alone in the world. I will wait for you, and will marry nobody else.'

These are not the letters of a woman so much under the influence of her lover that she had got to obey him whether she liked it or not. She even suggested that she had been hypnotised by Clark, but all the hypnotism in the world would not have made her write, 'I have fully made up my mind to administer the liquid at dinner on the 27th in mulligatawy soup, which will disguise the taste. Thursday will be the best day to finish this dreadful business. Send me the liquid after disguising its taste, and trust me to do the rest.'

When she received the liquid Clark sent her she wrote, 'The liquid has arrived safely, and if it is God's will, He will make all our efforts come to a successful issue to-day. It is exceptionally hot, and just the weather for a heatstroke. This is really the crisis in both our lives.'

On the following day she wrote a hurried note. 'They have taken dear hubby to the hospital after a most dreadful night. He was in a raving delirium, and was quite unconscious.'

Two days later, after treatment at the hospital, we find her writing, 'I have had a great disappointment, but it is evidently God's will to spare my hubby's life. He is not going to die.'

It is difficult to understand the state of mind in which she was capable of such a mixture of blasphemy, cynicism, and hypocrisy. She was utterly incapable of straight thinking. One minute she was bemoaning the fact that her husband was not dead and the next crying out against seeing him in pain.

'This last attempt has been a dead failure. They have diagnosed hubby's case as heatstroke. Nobody has the slightest suspicion of the truth. If only I had foreseen all this trouble I should never have made such an attempt on his poor life, which has resulted in nothing but a cruel disappointment and the wrecking of his whole nervous system. I have been quite downhearted since the last attempt and failure, and have no hopes of being free in this world. Hubby is getting better, and you must reconcile yourself to losing me.'

On October 3rd Mr Fulham had decided to go to Agra, and his wife wrote and told Clark. He died there on October 11th, and three days later she wrote to her lover, 'I never felt so happy and blissful in my life.'

Yet, in the face of these remarkable letters which were read out at the trial, Mrs Fulham put in a statement in which she said among other things, 'I knew Clark four years ago. He frequently came to our house at Meerut, and fell in love with me. Clark was most friendly with my husband. He made me and my husband do whatever he wished, and won my affection completely from my husband. I believe Clark must have the power of hypnotism. I became a tool in his hands. . . . When Mr Fulham was dying he called out "Clark" in a loud voice. Mr Fulham also said, "Look after my wife and children," showing he trusted Clark to the last.'

By no stretch of imagination can Mrs Fulham, in the face of her damning letters, be said to have acted under any other influence than that of an overpowering desire to have Clark all to herself. If she were the tool she suggested she was in her statement, she was a very willing tool. She not only carried out the suggestions of her lover, but she made suggestions of her own for expediting matters, and when her husband still lingered on despite her efforts, expressed herself in the bitterest terms of disappointment.

The story of the night of the unhappy man's death in Agra was told in moving evidence by the dead man's daughter Kathleen, who was only ten years of age.

'Daddy became ill after dinner on the night he died,' she said. 'Before that he had been quite well. We had dinner in the garden and mother took the dinner out to him.'

Note how, even at the last, the two lovers worked together for their common object! Clark provided the fatal dose, and Mrs Fulham administered it!

'Afterwards,' continued Kathleen, 'Daddy complained of the heat and went to bed. Lieutenant Clark was there at the time. During their dinner I heard daddy call out to him from the bedroom. Mr Clark went to him and stayed three or four minutes.'

A moment later she burst into tears, and it was some time before she could finish her story, one which would have broken down anyone three times her age.

'Later in the evening daddy said he was going and then added, "Be good. God bless you." He asked me where mummy was, and then said, "Don't call her."

'When I left daddy I saw Mr Clark and mummy in the dining-room. Mr Clark took a red box from a shelf and took out a glass needle. He opened a paper he had got and poured some powder from it into a wineglass of water, and filled the needle from it. He then went into daddy's room and seemed to push the needle into daddy's heart and arm and shoulder. A minute afterwards daddy gave a funny gurgling noise. I went to his bedside wondering what was the matter and saw daddy was lying on his back and breathing very heavily. Mr Clark came in and felt daddy's heart. He went back almost immediately into the dining-room and said to mummy, "Gone."

'After that Mr Clarke went out on a bicycle and fetched Captain Dunn. When he arrived Mr Clark pretended he did not know daddy was dead and said he had brought Captain Dunn to see how he was.'

In reply to a pertinent question by the counsel for the prosecution, she said she did not see any tears in her mother's eyes on the night her father died, but she cried a little the next day when the coffin was closed.

Even Mrs Fulham had to observe the properties which the world demanded of a day-old widow, though two days afterwards she was writing to Clark that she had never felt so happy and blissful in all her life before!

At the trial it was proved that Clark had bought large quantities of drugs from Calcutta—gelsemium, atropine, cocaine and arsenic. He tried to explain away the large amounts he had bought by saying that he had had to use them in the course of his practice. He gave the names of patients for whom he had had to use gelsemium. This is a drug very rarely used in medicine. Its effect is to act as a depressant, making the patient feel very wretched. If taken in poisonous doses it slows and enfeebles the heart, makes breathing more difficult, and causes extreme weakness and partial paralysis. These were exactly the symptoms from which Mr Fulham was suffering when he was taken to the hospital at Meerut. These symptoms could easily be mistaken for those of heatstroke—and in fact they were. It is a significant fact that no antidote for the poison was known to Clark.

'It would be interesting,' said the counsel for the prosecution, 'to know what happened to those patients of the prisoner to whom gelsemium was administered.'

'I cannot tell you,' said Clark. 'One of them died after a short illness.' He did not say, however, which one.

Evidence was given that Clark, on his arrest, had in his possession a book on poisons. The pages dealing with the effects of cocaine, atropine, arsenic, and other drugs were heavily marked. Those dealing with the effects of arsenic, in fact, were underlined. The doctor who carried out the *post mortem* examination of Mr Fulham testified that he had died from repeated doses of arsenic, and that the symptoms described in Mrs Fulham's fatal letters were consistent with long-continued doses of arsenic.

Such was the evidence against the two accused in regard to the death of Mr Fulham. The evidence againt them for the murder of Mrs Clark was as dramatic. As with the case of one of the dead man's children, one of the murdered woman's children gave evidence which was damning against the father. That was Harry Clark, the eldest son of Clark. The latter tried to discount the evidence before it was given.

'All my children are against me,' he declared. 'They have been so for years. I never instigated anyone to murder my wife.'

'My father was in the habit of visiting Mrs Fulham at Meerut,' said Harry Clark. 'My parents were far from being happy together. My father did not care for the family at all, and had no love for mother. I doubt whether he had any love for any of us either. My father was always more attentive to other ladies than to my mother. She was of a very quiet disposition, and not at all quarrelsome. She never neglected her household duties. My father has struck her in my presence. She told me that she was afraid she would be poisoned.'

Other witnesses gave evidence that Clark spoke of his wife in the most objectionable terms, and had said on more than one occasion that he would like to get rid of her.

Mrs Clark had little doubt, indeed, that her husband would poison her if he got the chance. She kept a diary and among the entries in it were the following:

'Why is Clark always so angry with me and the children? Everyone of my friends in Agra is telling me that Mrs Fulham has been living with my husband as his wife even while Mr Fulham was alive.

'My cook must have poisoned me. I was very bad, as the ward servant's wife had exercised witchcraft on me.

'We brought a good cook from Delhi, but he soon ran away, saying that Clark gave him three white powders to give in tea, and told him that if he did not give them he would kill him.

'Last month I was very ill with vomiting, as the cook had put something in the tea. I am perfectly sick and tired of living with Clark.

What will he do with all his money? Give it to Mrs Fulham or leave it to the children?'

That there was good ground for the unhappy woman's suspicion that she was being poisoned was proved in evidence by one of Clarke's daughters, who related how her mother had been very ill after drinking tea. His son had taken some powders which Clark had been giving to his wife and asked another doctor about them.

The doctor told him that the powder was a slow poison. Clark's son related that one night while they were having dinner his mother had only eaten two spoonfuls of rice when she was taken ill. His father was not at home that night for dinner. The native servant who had seved his mother was one of those who was arrested for murdering her, and he confessed that he had been given powders by Clark to put in Mrs Clark's food.

Maud Clark, a daughter of Clark, was also called upon to give evidence against her father. One of the most terrible features of this case was the evidence of the children of the accused, evidence which was never in their favour. It was Maud who was in the house when her mother was killed.

She related that her mother had strongly objected to her father's association with Mrs Fulham and they were always quarrelling about it.

'Once,' she said, 'mother saw a letter from Mrs Fulham to her father and returned it to the postman unopened. She told me that she was sure father was trying to poison her, and that very morning she complained that the tea tasted funny. My tea was all right,' added the witness.

She was asked to relate exactly what happened on the night of her mother's death.

'Father left the house between five and six o'clock and warned mother to be careful as there were thieves about. I was awakened about midnight by my mother screaming, and I saw a native with a stick in his hand by my mother's bed. She was bleeding, and I did what I could to help her. When father came in he said to mother, "Lovie, lovie speak! What has happened?" I asked him why he had not returned until so late, as he usually came in at ten o'clock, and he told me that he had been to see a friend at the Agra cantonment, but he did not say who it was. He never asked her what had happened that night.'

It came out in evidence that the first person Clark told of his wife's death was Mrs Fulham. He was with Mrs Fulham while his hired native assassins were removing the last obstacle. She must, indeed, when she heard the news, have never 'Felt more blissful and happy.'

But Mrs Fulham's love was not the kind to last. When her own neck was in danger she offered to turn King's evidence against her lover, but the judge refused to allow her to do so. She was asked in the witness-box if she were still prepared to marry Clark and she promptly replied, 'No.' When her offer to turn King's evidence was refused she made an attempt to prove that she was more sinned against than sinning, but her letters were too incriminating for her to be believed.

Clark came out of the ordeal much better. Inhuman though he had been, he did not, at any rate, try to put any of the blame on the woman for whom he had risked everything. When the case for the prosecution was closed Clark evidently realised that his chances of being found 'Not Guilty' were negligible.

'The letters which have been read in Court,' said the judge, 'tend to show that Mrs Fulham systematically administered poison to her husband under your directions from April 20th, 1911. What explanation have you to give?'

It was then that Clark took the dramatic and final step. While the judge had been speaking he seemed to lose the coolness he had hitherto displayed in the dock. He was very agitated for a while and then he pulled himself together.

'I am wholly and solely to blame,' he declared. 'Mrs Fulham was acting under my directions. I sent the drugs, and she gave them. She acted under my influence. She is not to blame.'

'You gave Mr Fulham injections on the night of his death,' said the judge.

'Yes. At first I intended making him sick by giving him small doses, so that he would have to leave the country. The last dose made him very ill. I was sorry for his condition. That is why I killed him. I simply administered four drams of antipyrin before dinner and this killed him. The injections I gave him after dinner were ether, digitalis, and strychnine, but the dose was too small to counteract the effects of the antipyrin. I gave him antipyrin because Fulham was a wreck and I wanted to finish him off. The injections were given only on the pretence of doing something for him. I knew they would not do any good.'

'I understand,' said the judge. 'You intended to kill him. Did you kill him?'

'Yes. I took pity on his condition.'

Although her counsel made a powerful pleas for Mrs Fulham on the grounds that she had been completely under the influence of her paramour, it took the jury exactly ten minutes to find her guilty.

Medical evidence was called to prove that she was expecting a child and her sentence was commuted to penal servitude for life. Following their trial, there came that of the four Hindus who had murdered Mrs Clark under her husband's orders. One turned King's evidence and the other three were found guilty and sentenced to death. Clark was executed at Allahabad on March 26th, 1913, and his three Hindu servants a week later.

Mrs Fulham, whose baby boy was born in prison, died ten months after its birth. It was the irony of fate that she died as the results of a heatstroke.

EDMUND L. PEARSON
Nineteen Dandelions

There was a tennis party, and Major Armstrong was skipping about the court, playing in a set of doubles. He was correctly and spotlessly dressed in flannels, and was as fussy and polite as usual.

Suddenly a figure of gloom appeared at the sidelines, and Mrs Armstrong's voice boomed out:

'Come, Herbert! It's six o'clock—how can you expect the servants to be punctual, if the master is late for dinner?'

Now, the little Major, in obeying his wife, was a perfect lamb. So he tucked his racquet under his arm, apologized to his astonished partner and opponents, and trotted away behind Mrs Armstrong—who was a good six inches taller than himself.

Of course, the match was ruined for the three remaining players. They stood staring for a moment, until they were reminded that others were waiting for the court. Then they moved resentfully off, and sat down with the spectators—who were smiling and whispering. The only ones who were much astonished were those who did not know the Armstrongs very well.

Almost everybody in the town of Hay did know the Armstrongs. The Major was pretty well liked, and he was even courted by some who thought it wise to keep on good terms with him. Mrs Armstrong was respected, and, moreover, was probably admired by ladies who approved of her system of keeping a husband under strict discipline.

She gazed forbiddingly from behind steel-rimmed spectacles. She was a martyr to frail health—nothing much the matter with her. Her ideas of etiquette were firm; she even let young Mr Martin, the lawyer, feel her disapproval for coming to one of her tea parties in flannel trousers and a sports coat. Martin was Major Armstrong's brother lawyer, and for that reason, if for no other, had been treated by the older man with courtesy.

But to Mrs Armstrong, her husband's military rank, his university education, and his position as Clerk of Courts were matters of importance. You did not attend Mrs Armstrong's tea parties in tennis clothes any more than you would try to get into Buckingham Palace in shirt sleeves.

Tennis seemed to get small consideration from Mrs Armstrong. It had no claims on her good manners. On another occasion she broke up the Major's game by reminding him that this was his 'bath night.'

You could not fail to notice Major Armstrong. When you talked with him, you were constantly aware of his blue eyes. Very blue they were—light blue—someone said they were the colour of forget-me-nots. And they shone, as with a light, while he looked straight at you, and talked—at great length—about himself and his affairs. It is not true that all murderers have blue eyes, but it is true that they have been a noticeable feature in a number of men whose careers were full of danger to people about them.

The Major was small and very dapper. He weighed ninety-eight pounds. He was neatly made, and carried himself so well—perhaps as a result of military training—that he did not seem little until he stood near someone of ordinary height.

His dress and adornment expressed his personality, for it was of a kind only to be described as 'natty.' He wore a boutonnière; his straw-coloured moustache was waxed at the ends; his collars and cravats were a joy to the haberdasher. His glasses—behind which glittered those eyes of heaven's blue—were of the *pince-nez* variety, and I think they were secured by a slender gold chain and a gold hook which encircled his right ear.

He was concerned with tiny details and fond of dickering over trifling matters of business, and playing with mechanical gadgets. Yet this little henpecked man, with his gold eyeglasses and his nice manners, became a terror in the community. People were afraid to eat or drink in his presence, and two of his neighbours—a man and wife—lay awake at night, fairly trembling at the thought of the blue-eyed Major.

Most of us think of murder as something far distant. It happens among gunmen or gangsters, generally among people a long way off. Certainly, not among our neighbours; not on our own street. If we know anything about life in a small town, it is hard to imagine that someone whom the neighbours respect is, as a matter of fact, as dangerous as a rattlesnake. That while he is talking to you, he may be deciding that you will be the next on his list. That if he offers you a cup of tea or if he invites you to dinner you will accept at your peril.

'No,' we say, 'that does not happen in our town.'

And that is what the people of the town of Hay would have said until they found out about Major Armstrong. Hay is a little place, on the border of England and Wales, and it had no more respectable citizen than the Major.

He was Master of Arts of Cambridge University, and held the King's commission in the Great War. He had not dropped his military title, but insisted on being addressed as Major. His law firm had borne the quaint name of Cheese and Armstrong, but now Mr Cheese was dead. The Major had only one rival for the legal business of the whole region. This was Mr Martin.

Armstrong may have looked back upon the years of the war with longing. Living with Mrs Armstrong was a little like being married to the president of the W.C.T.U., the general director of the Anti-Tobacco Society, and the author of an encyclopedia of etiquette, all at once.

She was a rigid teetotaler; therefore her husband must not drink wine or spirits. When they dined out, and the servant prepared to fill Armstrong's glass, the Major would be given no chance to decline for himself. From the other end of the table, Mrs Armstrong's stentorian voice would be heard:

'No wine for the Major!'

Mrs Armstrong played the piano with acid correctness, and she disapproved of tobacco. The Major actually smuggled his pipe into his pocket, or tossed his cigar over a hedge—like a schoolboy caught by the master—if he met his wife coming along the street. In his own home, there was one room only in which she permitted him to indulge in the foul practice of smoking.

The Major must have been one of those men who read with amusement the resolutely gloomy novels which so many literary men have written about the horrors of war, the dreadful life of camp and trench. A career under military regulations must have seemed lightsome and free as compared with the way he was kept goose-stepping at home.

His house was a pleasant villa called 'Mayfield,' and here he had a number of enemies. They were dandelions. He had a fine lawn—what Mr Kipling called a mint-sauce lawn—and he had also a garden. The lawn was infested with dandelions, and the Major hated them. He used to come out and glare at the weeds, marring his closely mown turf. Then he would sigh heavily, go downtown, and order five more gallons of weed-killer. Sometimes, for variety, he would buy half a pound of arsenic. He even bought arsenic in the winter, which was a curious time to prepare for dandelions. Still, it is always well to be ready for the changing seasons. Probably he murmured, 'If Winter comes, can Spring be far behind?'

He had a little squirt-gun, a delightfully delicate thing, with a tiny nozzle. This was for punishing dandelions. You see, if your lawn is like a putting green, to dig up a dandelion makes a nasty hole. But if you fill a squirt-gun with powdered arsenic, and then tiptoe gently up to the dandelion when it is off its guard, insert the nozzle near the root, and then—quick—press the plunger, why the dandelion begins to peak and pine, and pretty soon it passes away altogether. Without harming the grass.

The Major had great fun with his dandelion destroyer.

About this time—it was in July, 1920—Mrs Armstrong made a new will. She had some property, which had been willed in part to her children, and in part to her husband. Now, another will was made—all in the Major's handwriting, and rather irregularly witnessed. The whole property now was to go to her husband.

In August, the dandelions began to get bold and mischievous once more, and the Major resolutely went out and got three cans of poisoned weed-killer. He would show 'em!

In the same month, Mrs Armstrong's health declined. She had obscure complaints, and it was said she was not altogether right in her mind. Rheumatism, it is true, she had had for years. But these new troubles were serious, and, from now on, the poor lady is entitled to sympathy. Even the hardest-hearted tennis player or wine drinker must admit that. She was frightfully sick, and in the midst of it all was certified as insane, and carried off to a private asylum. Her doctors and her sister agreed that this was wise. Nobody could be more attentive—no one could, to all appearances, be a more dutiful husband than the little Major.

At the asylum, she seemed slowly to get better, mentally and physically. By January she had made such a recovery as to be able to come home. It was just before her return that the Major bought, in midwinter, the half-pound of arsenic. Still thinking of his lawn, and the accursed dandelions!

Mrs Armstrong's improvement, so marked while she was away, did not continue when she was back at 'Mayfield.' Soon she was ill again, and a nurse was called in. The delusions returned; she heard people walking about the house. She could take or retain no food, and spent most of the time in bed, slowly getting feebler.

The Major was solicitous, often coming home from his office in the middle of the day, and sometimes relieving the nurse on watch. This was not the dandelion season; he had no present foes in the garden or on the lawn, and the squirt-gun, presumably, was put away.

At last, late in February, after weeks of distressing sickness, Mrs Amstrong died. Dr Hinckes, the local physician, and a good one, certified that she had a complication of diseases. She was buried in the churchyard. Only a few friends came to the funeral; they noticed that the widower seemed calm. In fact, while the coffin was being brought down, he was chatting with one of the other mourners about fishing rights.

Next Sunday his grief was more apparent. At the church they held a kind of memorial service for the late parishioner, and Major Armstrong, himself, read the lesson, 'with great eloquence and feeling.'

Winter vanished, and the warmer days arrived. Dandelions began to threaten the lawn at 'Mayfield' and the Major planned his spring offensive. He had been away for a few weeks, for rest and change of scene, and during these holidays renewed his wartime acquaintance with the mysterious lady known only as 'Mrs———.' After he got back to Hay, he gave little dinner parties, mostly for gentlemen. Wine was no longer forbidden. From one of these dinners, a guest—the local inspector of taxes—went home rather ill, and had a bad night.

It is a curious thing about the poisoner: one success almost always makes him try again. The crime for which a poisoner is arrested is usually not his first, nor even his second. The employment of poison gives a sense of power; a feeling which seems to make the poisoner say to himself:

'Nobody knows what a weapon I have. People, if they recognized my power, would respect me more—and fear me more.'

Poison is, therefore, frequently the weapon of quiet, furtive people; of small, inoffensive-appearing persons; of meek-looking women; of men who are a little effeminate, a bit sly in manner.

The Major's next experiment may have been upon Mr Davies, from the neighbouring city of Hereford. He had a small business controversy with Major Armstrong, and came to Hay to discuss it. The Major invited him to his house to tea. How the business was settled I do not know, but Mr Davies no sooner got home than he had a very bad pain. He called the doctor, and they operated for appendicitis. When the certificate came to be signed, it appeared that Mr Davies had had acute appendicitis, resulting in peritonitis, which, in turn, resulted in death.

Summer was a-coming in. 'Mrs——' appeared on the scene again. She made a brief visit to 'Mayfield,' and seems to have been considering a proposal of marriage. The Major showed her his garden and lawn, and perhaps told her of his triumphs over the dandelions. It was her great good luck that she took some time to consider whether she wished to become the bride of this man.

The legal business meanwhile was improving, with nobody but the friendly Mr Martin to dispute it, or to appear on the opposite side in litigation. Mr Martin, who was a wounded veteran of the war, had persuaded a young lady to marry him. He brought his bride to the town of Hay, where they set up housekeeping. In the late summer, they received a package by mail; a present of some chocolates. There was no name enclosed, and they mildly wondered who sent them.

There are still people who receive these strange gifts, from nobody in particular, and who go right ahead and eat them. Others let them stay around till someone else tastes them. The Martins did not care for chocolates, but put them in a dish and brought them out at a dinner party. Someone took a bite, and this someone was beastly sick. Afterwards—when many other things had happened—the remaining chocolates were found and examined. On the under side of a number of them there was a small hole, as though a tiny nozzle had been inserted. And in these chocolates there was a little bit of arsenic.

Mr Martin and the Major were representing the parties to a business deal—a sale of land. The Major's client did not complete the contract and Martin had to press him, and, after a year's delay, to threaten to declare the contract broken and demand return of the deposits. The Major was agitated and kept pleading for more time. In October, after postponements, Martin's client finally refused to go on with the sale, and insisted that the deposits be returned.

Major Armstrong's remedy for this was tea. There is something about tea conductive to friendliness, and it seemed to him that these troubles would clear up, if he could only get the other lawyer looking at him across a tea table. You must remember that at this time nobody had examined the chocolates, and that the deaths and illnesses which had occurred were attributed to various diseases.

After repeated invitations, Mr Martin did go, late one afternoon, to 'Mayfield,' where his soft-spoken little host received him with smiling courtesy. The two lawyers' offices were directly opposite each other, on the business street of the town, but the Major had gone home first—to see that everything was prepared and pleasant.

There was tea, and there was bread and butter, and there was bread with currants in it, and there were buttered scones. The two men did not discuss legal business at all, except in a general way, and the question of the land contract did not come up. But very soon after the tea was poured, the Major—for a man so fussy and so well-mannered—did a strange thing. He reached across and picked up a buttered scone, which he put on Mr Martin's plate with the remark:

'Please excuse fingers.'

Mr Martin ate the scone; then he had some currant bread, smoked a cigarette, talked a while and went home. He found himself with poor appetite for dinner, although he ate a little. In the evening he tried to do some work, dictating to a secretary, but had to give it up. He became, first, very uncomfortable, and then, for twenty-four hours, violently sick. The same doctor who had attended Mrs Armstrong was his physician.

Martin remembered the urgent invitations to tea; he recalled the scene; and, during the week that followed, as he slowly returned to health, he resolved to deny himself the pleasure of any further teas with the Major. He had a father-in-law who was a chemist, and this gentleman thought that he recognized something about the symptoms of his son-in-law's illness. He insisted upon an analysis. When this revealed the presence of arsenic, both of them, as well as the doctor, thought it time to communicate with the government.

The officials did not hurry; they agreed that things were suspicious, but nothing more than suspicious. The doctor began to remember peculiar circumstances of Mrs Armstrong's last illness. And all of them warned Mr Martin not to accept any more treats at 'Mayfield.'

It was good advice, even if not needed. But it was hard advice to follow. Major Armstrong began to talk about tea once more. He called on his brother lawyer, as soon as he returned to work; commiserated him upon his illness, and playfully recalled that he had warned him against lack of exercise. In the Major's opinion, Mr Martin was taking too little exercise. He ought to walk more, and use his motor car less.

'And it may seem a curious thing to say,' added Major Armstrong, 'but I fear you will have another attack just like that one!'

Mr Martin looked at him, and almost turned green. He hoped not.

'And now, old man,' pursued the affable Major, 'we must have another talk about that sale. My clients have a proposal to make. Come to tea to-morrow.'

Mr Martin was sorry. He had an engagement. No, positively. He could not come.

'Oh, very well,' returned Armstrong.

But next day he was back again—this time by telephone.

'Come in to tea, won't you?'

'Sorry,' said the terrified Martin, 'not taking any tea today.'

Next day the business really did require a settlement, and Martin realized that he must talk with his neighbour.

'Will you come over to tea, this afternoon?' telephoned the Major.

'No,' was the reply. 'I can't come to tea. But I will look in afterwards—around six o'clock.'

But this wouldn't do. There was something about this contract that could be settled only over the teacups.

'Well, never mind,' the Major replied, 'come to tea tomorrow.'

Then it occurred to Armstrong that taking your tea in your office is a good English custom. Perhaps Martin didn't like to go so far as 'Mayfield.' The Major set up a tea caddy, cups and spoons in his office, had his housekeeper send down some scones, and instructed one of his clerks to order some bread and cake from the restaurant nearby.

'I tell you what,' said he, 'we'll have tea in my office. Come over about half-past four.'

Mr Martin could only stammer. He had run out of excuses. He and his wife were thoroughly agitated now; they saw the Major's gleaming blue eyes everywhere. They actually took turns in keeping awake all night; one of them on guard while the other slept. Evidently they expected the Major to come climbing up the wistaria vine, armed with an arsenic bottle.

That afternoon the telephone rang again.

'Where are you?' came the Major's voice. 'The tea is spoiling; been waiting half an hour.'

'Oh, I've had my tea,' said the wretched man. 'Had it here in my office.'

After this, Martin—while the police investigated—was reduced to bringing tea into his own office and hastily gulping it.

I have wondered why he didn't accept someday; go over, and give Major Armstrong every opportunity to prepare the dishes; take them from his hands, then turn on him, and say:

'Oh, Major, I couldn't think of taking these. Look, this cup of tea, so nice and hot! And this lovely buttered bun! I want *you* to have these!'

And back the little viper right into a corner with the stuff.

But this might have given the show away, and ruined Scotland Yard's investigations. The Major, so far, had the whip hand, and he knew it. Martin was frightened. When the tea invitations ceased at last, and Armstrong began to ask Mr and Mrs Martin to dinner, the younger lawyer was desperate.

All this time Scotland Yard was working on the case, and telling Martin to hold out a little longer. It was a serious thing to arrest such an important and respectable person as the Major, and to accuse him of the extraordinary offense of trying to murder a fellow lawyer with a poisoned scone. It would not do to make a mistake.

Finally, a detective inspector came down from London, and, to the utter amazement of everyone—except the Martins, and one or two others—arrested the Major for attempted murder.

At the same time—a dark winter night—strange men appeared in the town and strange lights were seen in the churchyard. England's famous pathologist, Sir Bernard Spilsbury, and his aides were exhuming the body of Mrs Armstrong.

As soon as the coffin was opened, all the doctors knew, by the extraordinary manner in which the body was preserved, that this was probably a death by arsenic. And the autopsy revealed the largest amount of that poison ever found in such circumstances.

It was for murder, the murder of his wife, that the Major was tried. He was defended by one of the great criminal lawyers of the day, Sir Henry Curtis Bennett, who did his best to show that Mrs Armstrong—utterly helpless at the time—might have arisen from bed, and taken the poison herself.

Mr Martin's story of the tea party was admitted as evidence, and the judge (Lord Darling) took a vigorous part in cross-examining the prisoner. In the United States, it is probable that the Major's lawyers would have succeeded in excluding Martin's evidence, and the prisoner would have escaped. The theory of Mrs Armstrong's suicide might have seemed stronger if her husband had not been revealed as a systematic poisoner.

Major Armstrong sat bolt upright in court, calm and attentive—staring, with his pale blue eyes, straight ahead. While he was on the witness stand, he and the judge had a long verbal duel, conducted with icy politeness. The Major described how he had made up twenty little packets of arsenic, each containing a deadly dose for a dandelion.

It was also, the judge pointed out, a deadly dose for a human being, was it not?

And he had used nineteen of these packets on nineteen dandelions. As the Major described the process, in his precise voice, you could almost see the graves of the nineteen dandelions.

And there was one little packet left over (as the judge observed) and it was found in his pocket, when he was arrested, in December.

The jury—most of them farmers—were capable of noting that in December the dandelion season is practically over.

A year or two later, that graceful writer, Mr Filson Young, visited the town of Hay, and sat on the lawn at 'Mayfield.' The dandelions, he says, were thicker than ever.

They had triumphed. The Major was far away. He was not even lying in that churchyard whither he had sent one, or two, or how many others? For the concluding words of the dread sentence of the law in England are:

'. . . and that you be there hanged by the neck until you be dead; that your body be buried within the precincts of the prison in which you shall last be confined; and may the Lord have mercy on your soul.'

And the chaplain, standing behind the judges, replies:

'Amen!'

JUDGE GERALD SPARROW
A Psychopathic Murderer

1972 was a vintage year for those who are fascinated by poisoners, by murderers whose minds are 'disturbed', by compulsive killing and by the whole disputed area of madness and the Law. It was the year in which Graham Frederick Young was sentenced at St Albans Crown Court to life imprisonment for murdering Mr Robert Egle, head storeman at Hadlands Laboratories, Mr Frederick Biggs of Chipperfield, and of attempting to murder David John Price Tilson, and Jethro Batt, as well as administering poison to Ronald Hewitt and Diana Smart.

The case created a public uproar not only because this dangerous psychopath had been using his work mates as guinea pigs in poison experiments, but because the whole sordid and dreadful affair could have been avoided if anyone had paid the slightest attention to what Mr Justice Melford Stevenson had said ten years earlier, in 1962, when Young had been charged with poisoning his father and sister. The Judge had sent Young to Broadmoor Criminal Lunatic Asylum with the most positive recommendation that he should not be released for 15 years without the Home Secretary's consent. Young in fact was released, in February 1971, nine years later, and within three months had started a mad poisoning spree with the dreadful results that ended in his second trial.

Apart from the fact that he was released far too soon the authorities—who acted of course on medical advice—might have been warned by the fact that Young, even as a boy of fourteen, was administering poison to relations, friends, and acquaintances as opportunity offered in a motiveless way. This was the real hallmark of the mad, compulsive killer. He was not actuated by hate, or greed, or sexual desire, in his abnormal and deranged mind he was a chemical genius and those privileged to aid him in his experiments with poisons by becoming his victims were merely 'interesting' in so far as they provided him with more knowledge of various types of poison, details of lethal doses, and the time it took the 'subject' to die. This was what had made Mr Justice Stevenson write his awful warning. 'Such people are always dangerous and are adept at concealing their mad compulsion which may never be wholly cured.'

However, Home Secretaries these days are nothing if not fashionable and Mr Justice Eveleigh made no comment when he passed the sentence of life imprisonment. There was in fact no need for comment. The whole dreadful sequence of events had been fully reported in the Press and once again we were indebted to detailed and accurate reporting of the case and its bizarre history for the measures which at last the authorities felt impelled to take in order to prevent, if they could, a recurrence of this tragedy.

The story of Graham Frederick Young I find totally fascinating because it shows the madness of a man beginning to show itself in the child, and that insanity never alters basically while he grows up. Young was a compulsive and cunning poisoner as a boy. He remained a compulsive and cunning poisoner as a man.

In July 1962 Young was top chemistry pupil at John Kelly Secondary School, Willesden. His knowledge of poisons was phenomenal. His friends were chemists from whom by forged prescriptions he obtained poisons. He started in a simple way by putting antimony in a cream biscuit and giving it to his best school friend, John Williams. He laced his sister's tea with belladonna. He sprinkled his father's food with an antimony 'dressing.' He had a perfectly normal family life. His father and sister were good to him. He owed them no grudge. Fortunately an alert science master caught this brilliant pupil with an authorised poison and reported the matter which led to his arrest. Had it not been for this Frederick Young might well have been a juvenile murderer. As it was his three victims, after being very ill, recovered.

When detectives searched Young's room they found the same kind of books that Ian Brady the Moor murderer had in his possession. There was the same dedication to Hitler, but whereas Brady worshipped the cult of de Sade, this fourteen-year-old boy had a whole library on poison—and on poisoners. They were his heroes. William Palmer, Pritchard, George Chapman, right down to Mrs Merryfield who was very properly hanged in 1953 at a time when the good, clean crack of the rope was still putting the fear of God into killers and forcing the robbers to leave their guns at home.

There was no doubt that Young was a very bright boy indeed. The chemists he consorted with thought of him as a prodigy and a 'chemical genius.' Perhaps he was, but it was genius horrible and lethally perverted.

Young had ten shillings a week pocket money and out of this slender income he managed to build up a formidable library on poisons. He read every book he acquired avidly so that the mind of this schoolboy was filled with the idea of poison to the exclusion of all else. It was the only subject that really interested him. It was his life.

At his first trial this good-looking schoolboy with his curly chestnut hair admitted the charges and gave no explanation.

At this trial the Judge heard the evidence of Dr Christopher Fysh, chief Medical Officer of the remand centre where Young had been placed. Dr Fysh said that Young was suffering from 'A psychopathic disorder'. Asked by the Judge whether he was likely to repeat this kind of crime, Dr Fysh, who seems to have been a practical as well as an experienced doctor, said; 'I think it is extremely likely.' Again this dreadful warning was apparently forgotten or overruled with the dreadful results that led to the second trial.

The life that Young led in Broadmoor may come as a surprise to readers who have been left behind in the great swing to liberalism in prison administration; 'Young's prolific reading made him well-informed. He had access to all daily and Sunday newspapers. He was able to borrow books—on poison of course, from Berkshire County Council's mobile library. He could out-talk most of the inmates and nurses on a variety of subjects and was especially brilliant on medical matters and poisons.

From 7 am daily he was free to do as he liked, although he spent most of his time reading in his room. However, as he grew up he did grow a Hitler-type moustache and brushed his hair across his forehead even making himself a Swastika emblem. He watched television in the 'common room'—connoisseurs of phraseology will notice the University nomenclature—and radio in his room was allowed after he had become a parole patient for good behaviour. He kept and carefully tended a budgerigar. This bird seems to have suffered no ill effects and in the companionship between the boy and the bird we glimpse perhaps the only sight of sanity in the story of Graham Young. He grew deadly nightshade in the garden and extracted belladonna from it. He put sugar-soap in the patient's tea as a joke which was not appreciated.

Not a bad life, really. No expense, no worry, some companionship, time for study and assured privacy. No freedom, but no worries.

Perhaps the weirdest escapade of this extraordinary boy was to devise a way of getting drunk without alcohol which was forbidden. Young and his small circle used carbon monoxide taken from a gas automatic lighter. The flame was extinguished and the escaping gas was charged into the tea and milk. It was very intoxicating. Several drunken parties seem to have taken place in the common room. Obviously Young had a most ingenious mind.

Throughout his time at Broadmoor he made no special secret of the fact that he was fascinated by murder preferably by poison but not exclusively. He was an admirer of Christie, the horror killer of Rillington Place and knew every detail of the crimes that Christie committed. He even knew how many layers of wallpaper Christie had used to cover his foul crimes . . .

Mr Geoffrey Foster of Hadlands, Young's employer, described him as above average intelligence, but Mr Foster would never have employed him had he known of Young's Broadmoor record. This was suppressed to enable him to be 'rehabilitated' in a good job and, as the authorities explained, to ensure that he would rejoin normal society. There was of course never any chance of Graham Young rejoining normal society. Putting aside all the lawyers' jargon and all their definitions of insanity, and setting aside the medical 'scientific' approaches, Young was as mad as a hatter, and he revealed his madness most in the extraordinary cunning he showed in conning the Broadmoor doctors that he was totally cured when in reality his insanity had grown with the years.

Dr Edgar Unwin was responsible for Young under the medical superintendent Dr Patrick McGrath. Young, who could have the most winning manner if he chose, seems to have fooled both these very experienced doctors, Dr Unwin being a psychiatrist of repute, and Dr Unwin an expert in his field of medicine.

Dr Unwin in recommending Young to a Training centre at Slough before he got his job with Hadlands wrote: 'This man has suffered a deep-going personality disorder necessitating hospitalisation throughout his adolescence. . . . He has however made an extremely full recovery and is now entirely fit for discharge—his sole disability now being the need to catch up his lost time.'

It is easy to be wise after the event. Dr Unwin made a mistake. It may well be that Young would have deceived any psychiatrist such was his gift for making a good impression. When Hadlands had agreed to employ him the Slough Training Centre were equally enthusiastic about their trainee. No mention was made of Broadmoor by anyone. That was a thing of the past, A letter of thanks that Young wrote to Mr Foster shows how tactful and pleasing Young could be:

'Dear Mr Foster,

Thank you for your letter of the 26th instant offering me the job of assistant store keeper.

I am pleased to accept your offer and will therefore report for work on Monday the 10th of May at 8.30 am.

May I take this opportunity of expressing my gratitude to you for offering me this position notwithstanding my previous infirmity as communicated to you by the placing officer.

I shall endeavour to justify your faith in me by performing my duties in an efficient and competent manner.

Until Monday week, I am,
Yours faithfully,
Graham Young.'

It is just right, flawless. The little hurdle of the 'previous infirmity' is lightly touched on as a thing of the past, all the more reason for gratitude and faithful service to justify his employers faith in him. It is a polite letter but not servile, even friendly, and it is the letter of an educated and intelligent man who knew exactly what to say and how to express it.

The newspapers went to town on the story of Graham Young suggesting that there had been negligence or at least dire mistakes. I disagree. I think that everyone from the Home Secretary and his advisers to the Hadlands Director, the staff at the training centre, and the Broadmoor doctors, were taken for a ride by a psychopath of exceptional cunning and address, capable of ingratiating himself with the able, experienced and compassionate men who were deceived by cleverly contrived symptoms of sanity and a balanced, moderate approach which Graham Young could invoke at will. He was a consummate actor. He was insane only about murder. He was otherwise not only normal but extremely clever. His work at the training centre had been exemplary. Those in charge of him did not doubt for a moment that so able and industrious a young man would make good.

So the scene seemed to be set for success and there was confidence at Hadlands that the new man in the store was a very lucky find indeed. Young began working with Robert Egle, the chief store keeper, Mr Biggs, and Mr Hewitt.

Mr Egle was the first to go. The doctors never thought for one moment he had been poisoned. He was cremated. Young had killed him with thallium, a little known drug which Young had studied for ten years. As other members of the staff either died or were terribly ill without reason suspicion grew until detectives were called in and searched Young's room. Experienced policemen as they were they had never seen anything like it. There was a whole library on poison and poisoners. There were some very odd drawings of two hands administering poison to a victim. There were Nazi relics and literature. A favourite decorative theme of the room was a skull and crossbones.

Even with all this Young was able to play cat and mouse with the doctors who were called in. He even got himself appointed firm representative at the funeral of Mr Egle . . . It is of course common for murderers to obtain some sexual satisfaction from attending their victim's funeral but there is no evidence of sexuality in the record of this macabre man.

Eventually as sickness increased in Hadlands it became known as 'the Bovington bug.' It was dreaded. Everyone feared that they might catch it.

So we have the extraordinary picture of a happy and well-ordered firm of moderate size—there were about eighty employees—reduced to tension and suspicion because they felt themselves haunted by an unspecified disease that might strike anyone down at any moment.

Graham Young made the most discreet but painstaking enquiries as to the condition of those struck down with the 'Bovington bug'. He was genuinely absorbed in the reaction to the poisons which he had administered. Whether the victim lived or died seemed unimportant. When Mr Briggs perished, Young who seems to have liked him said, 'Dear old Fred. I'm so sorry.'

Thallium is tasteless and odourless. Graham Young knew his poisons.

A Committee was appointed under the amiable chairmanship of Lord Butler, the Master of Trinity College, Cambridge, to look into the whole matter and to recommend what—if anything—should be done.

SOURCES AND ACKNOWLEDGEMENTS

'Murder and the Mother Superior' (original title, 'Religious') by John Dunning, from *Murderous Women* (London: Hamlyn, 1983). Reproduced by permission of the author and David Bolt Associates.

'The Last of Mrs Maybrick' by Q. Patrick, from *Murder Cavalcade* (London: Hammond, Hammond & Company, 1953).

'Adelaide Bartlett' by Charles Franklin, from *World Famous Acquittals*. Reproduced by permission of The Hamlyn Publishing Group Limited.

'Murder for Murder's Sake', 'The Jekyll and Hyde of New York' and 'An Indian Holocaust' by John Lawrence, from *Extraordinary Crimes* (London: Sampson Low, Marston & Co., Ltd, n.d.).

'Poison in a Private School' and 'How Parsimony Hanged a Poisoner' by Harold Eaton, from *The Fifty Most Amazing Crimes of the Last 100 years* (London: Odhams Press Ltd, n.d.).

'The Long Island Borgia' by Leonard Gribble, from *Compelled to Kill* (London: Hutchinson Publishing Group 1977). Reproduced by permission of Lois Gribble.

'The Case of the Poisoned Bun' by Morris Markey, from *Fifty Strangest Stories Ever Told* (London: Odhams Press Ltd, n.d.).

'Madeleine Smith' by W.H. Williamson, from *Annals of Crime* (London: George Routledge & Sons, 1930). Reproduced by permission of Routledge & Kegan Paul Limited.

'Doctor Cream' and 'Nineteen Dandelions' by Edmund Pearson, from *Murder at Smutty Nose* (New York: The Sun Dial Press, Inc., 1938).

'The Hoop-La Murder Trial' by Sidney Horler, from *Malefactors' Row* (London: Hale, 1940).

'The Case of the Lady Who Lost Her Head' by Alan Hynd, from *Sleuths, Slayers and Swindlers* (London: Thomas Yoseloff Ltd, 1959). Reprinted by permission of Noel Hynd.

'The Angel-Makers of Nagzrev' by Bernard O'Donnell from *'The World's Worst Women'* (London: W.H. Allen & Co, 1953). Reproduced by permission of W.H. Allen & Company.

While every effort has been made to trace authors and copyright-holders, in some cases this has proved impossible. The publishers would be glad to hear from any such parties so that omissions can be rectified in future editions of the book.